# TREATING EATING DISORDERS WITH DBT

AF719623

# Treating Eating Disorders with DBT

## The MED-DBT Protocol

**Anita Federici**
**Lucene Wisniewski**

THE GUILFORD PRESS
New York London

Copyright © 2026 The Guilford Press
A Division of Guilford Publications, Inc.
*www.guilford.com*

All rights reserved

Except as indicated, no part of this book may be reproduced, translated, stored in a retrieval system, or transmitted, in any form or by any means, electronic, mechanical, photocopying, microfilming, recording, or otherwise, without written permission from the publisher.

Printed in the United States of America

This book is printed on acid-free paper.

For product and safety concerns within the EU, please contact *GPSR@taylorandfrancis.com,* Taylor & Francis Verlag GmbH, Kaufingerstraße 24, 80331 München, Germany.

Last digit is print number: 9 8 7 6 5 4 3 2 1

LIMITED DUPLICATION LICENSE

These materials are intended for use only by qualified mental health professionals.

The publisher grants to individual purchasers of this book nonassignable permission to reproduce all materials for which photocopying permission is specifically granted in a footnote. This license is limited to you, the individual purchaser, for personal use or use with clients. This license does not grant the right to reproduce these materials for resale, redistribution, electronic display, or any other purposes (including but not limited to books, pamphlets, articles, video or audio recordings, blogs, file-sharing sites, internet or intranet sites, and handouts or slides for lectures, workshops, or webinars, whether or not a fee is charged). Permission to reproduce these materials for these and any other purposes must be obtained in writing from the Permissions Department of Guilford Publications.

This publication is intended to provide helpful and informative material. It is not intended to diagnose, treat, cure, or prevent any health problem or condition, nor is it intended to replace the advice of a health professional. No action should be taken based solely on the contents of this book. Always consult your physician or qualified health care professional on any matters regarding your health and before adopting any suggestions in this book or drawing inferences from it.

The authors and publisher specifically disclaim all responsibility for any liability, loss, or risk, personal or otherwise, which is incurred as a consequence, directly or indirectly, from the use or application of any contents of this book.

Any and all product names referenced within this book are the trademarks of their respective owners. Always read all information provided by the manufacturers' product labels before using their products. The authors and publisher are not responsible for claims made by manufacturers.

Library of Congress Cataloging-in-Publication Data is available from the publisher

ISBN 978-1-4625-5848-3 (Hardcover)

*To our clients, our greatest teachers: you are the heart of MED-DBT.*

*This book is for our clients, who taught us that surviving is not enough and that building a life worth living is a revolutionary act.*

# About the Authors

**Anita Federici, PhD, CPsych,** is a clinical psychologist and founder of The Centre for Psychology and Emotion Regulation (*www.psychology-emotionregulation.ca*). She holds an Adjunct Faculty position at York University and is a Fellow of the Academy for Eating Disorders (AED). Internationally recognized for her expertise in eating disorders and dialectical behavior therapy, Dr Federici has delivered more than 400 lectures, workshops, and invited talks. She specializes in building sustainable, evidence-informed care systems through strategic consultation, implementation support, and team-based training for hospitals and organizations worldwide. Her work integrates clinical expertise and systems design to support the development of scalable, person-centered care pathways, particularly for underserved populations and clients with complex treatment needs. Dr. Federici's contributions have been featured at international conferences and published in peer-reviewed journals and edited book volumes.

**Lucene Wisniewski, PhD,** is Adjunct Assistant Professor of Psychological Sciences at Case Western Reserve University and founder and Chief Clinical Officer of the Center for Evidence Based Treatment (*www.cebtohio.com*), which offers therapy, training, and consultation in evidence-based approaches to a variety of mental health conditions via traditional and teletherapy platforms. She was appointed as Fellow of the AED for her leadership contributions to AED and the field of eating disorders. Dr. Wisniewski also has served on AED's board of directors and as co-chair of the Borderline Personality Disorder special interest group. In 2013, she received AED's Outstanding Clinician Award to acknowledge her commitment to providing the best solutions for those with eating disorders. In (including adapted versions in higher levels of care) shared particular characteristics, including the following:

1. Co-occurring personality disorders marked by impulsivity and pervasive problems with emotional regulation (Stice et al., 2008)
2. Recurrent suicidal and self-injurious behavior (Joiner, 2005)
3. High levels of perfectionism or rigidity (Hewitt et al., 1995)
4. Other severe co-occurring conditions such as major depressive disorder, anxiety disorders, obsessive–compulsive disorder (OCD), trauma, and substance use (Hambleton et al., 2022)
5. High levels of familial conflict or dysfunction (Eisler et al., 2000)

It was important for us to also recognize that the patients we wanted to help were often the ones excluded from major treatment outcome studies. Recurrent suicide and self-injury, substance use, use of multiple prescribed medications, and previous treatment trials are common exclusion criteria (Bulik et al., 2007; Eddy et al., 2017; Tchanturia et al., 2007, 2016). Our patients, then, are repeatedly expected to attend standard ED treatments *that were not designed for their unique needs* and are often labeled as resistant or unmotivated when they don't respond. The CBT-E and FBT manuals recognize the importance of assessing and managing these risks in individuals with eating disorders, but offer little to no direction with respect to how to treat multiple high-risk behaviors, co-occurring difficulties, or behaviors that interfere with treatment delivery.

In addition to client outcome data, we also observed that practitioners often disclosed to us that they felt frustrated, judgmental, burned out, and at a loss for how to help this group of patients (Burke et al., 2024; DeJong et al., 2012; Geller et al., 2012; Lubieniecki et al., 2024; Oliverio et al., 2022). As noted, instead of developing new care pathways, it seemed more common for our patients to be labeled as treatment resistant, unmotivated to change, manipulative, or attention-seeking. We were determined to do more for our patients. They needed something different: hope, a treatment plan, and providers who understood them. So we set out to develop MED-DBT.

## How to Use This Book

This book is the result of our ongoing commitment to treating individuals with multidiagnostic EDs—clients who have often been left out of traditional care pathways and research trials. We wrote this text for clinicians who are ready to do something different: to stay curious, to build deeper clinical insight, and to meet their clients with compassion and clarity. Whether you are new to DBT or an experienced provider, we hope this book offers both practical tools and guiding principles to support your work.

Organized in four sections, this manual will walk you through the foundational theories, treatment assumptions, and structure of the MED-DBT model. It also provides detailed strategies for each phase of treatment, including pretreatment, session planning, contingency management, and endings. We encourage you to read the book sequentially or to refer back to specific sections as you begin applying MED-DBT in your clinical work. Our goal is not only to support your clients in building a life worth living but also to help you find more sustainability and satisfaction in delivering care to this often underserved population.

All case examples are entirely fictional or composite, drawn from multiple clients and scenarios across clinical settings. No identifying details have been included.

# Acknowledgments

Writing this book has been a labor of energy, vision, collaboration, and shared passion over many years. We are profoundly grateful for the experience of coauthoring this work together, an experience built on mutual respect, creativity, countless hours of dialogue, and a shared commitment to building better care pathways for clients living with multidiagnostic eating disorders.

We extend our heartfelt thanks to Dr. Cynthia Bulik for her generous guidance in helping us accurately communicate the evolving science around genetics and metabolism, and to Dr. Mark Warren for helping us think through the intricate medical considerations that so often arise in this work.

We are especially indebted to the three incredible experts who took time out of their demanding schedules to review the book in full and provide invaluable feedback, strengthening both its structure and its spirit:

- Dr. Kelly Koerner, whose careful reading and insight elevated the clarity and integrity of the book,
- Dr. Pat Fallon, who offered thoughtful reflections that helped refine key ideas, and
- Dr. Melissa Freizinger, whose critical eye and encouragement were instrumental in shaping the final version.

We are immensely grateful to our publishing team at The Guilford Press. Special thanks to Kitty Moore, whose unwavering support and faith in this project made it possible, and to Katherine Sommer and Anna Bristow, whose exceptional editorial expertise and guidance shaped the manuscript with precision, care, and respect for the complexity of the work.

We also thank Jeremy Kaufmann and Madeline Herman for their assistance in refining early drafts and helping with the structural and referencing process.

Our clinical teams, The Centre for Psychology and Emotion Regulation (Ontario, Canada) and The Center for Evidence-Based Treatment (Ohio, U.S.A.), have been with us every step of the way. Their enthusiasm, feedback, and willingness to think through complex clinical examples with us made this work stronger than we could have achieved alone.

We are also grateful to colleagues Charlotte Thomas, Dr. Kimberly Claudat, and Shelly Hindle for their encouragement, research support, and steadfast belief in this project.

To our clients:

You are the heart of this book.

Your courage, your insistence that care pathways must evolve, your advocacy for treatments that recognize co-occurring difficulties, and your commitment to building lives worth recovering into—this book is for you and because of you.

We wish to acknowledge, with deepest reverence, Dr. Marsha M. Linehan, whose life, vision, and unwavering belief that "people in hell deserve to be helped" inspired not just DBT but the spirit of this entire work. A psychologist with lived experience, a radical thinker grounded equally in empirical science and deep spirituality, and a trailblazer who refused to give up on people others deemed "untreatable," Marsha Linehan taught the world a different way to see, to understand, and to care. It was her radical acceptance of suffering—not as a flaw but as part of the human condition—and her fierce commitment to building lives worth living, that shaped the framework within which MED-DBT was born.

Finally, thank you to all who believed in this project, who walked alongside us during its creation, and who continue to work toward a more compassionate, inclusive, and effective world of eating disorder care.

# Contents

Purchasers of this book can download and print additional copies of select materials at *www.guilford.com/federici-forms* for personal use or use with clients (see copyright page for details).

# Part I

# An Introduction to MED-DBT

MED-DBT is a comprehensive treatment designed for individuals with an eating disorder (ED) who also live with co-occurring psychiatric and physical conditions. Those with multidiagnostic issues often do not respond adequately to standard ED treatments and can be misunderstood as "treatment resistant" or lacking motivation to change. As you will learn, MED-DBT is a multimodel and intensive outpatient treatment that is delivered in phases to ensure informed consent, maximize collaboration, and build commitment between you and your client.

This first part of this book is designed to provide the history and development of MED-DBT with the aim of increasing your comfort in explaining the framework and rationale to potential clients. Your clients will want to know whether MED-DBT is a good fit for them and how it differs from other first-line ED treatments and other DBT for ED adaptations. In this part of the book, we outline the criteria for MED-DBT and provide guidelines to determine whether this treatment is suitable for your client. The assessment phase is the first step in MED-DBT and a necessary precursor to the pretreatment phase. Thus, this part includes the following:

- Chapter 1: The MED-DBT Program: Development and Foundations
- Chapter 2: Assessment for Treatment: Is MED-DBT a Good Fit for Your Client?

# 1

# The MED-DBT Program
## Development and Foundations

Eating disorders (EDs) are serious, multisystem illnesses characterized by persistent disturbances in eating behaviors, thoughts, sensory and perceptual experiences, and emotions that impact feeding behaviors, weight, and body image (Attia & Walsh, 2025; Brizzi et al., 2023; American Psychiatric Association, 2013). To live with an ED is to experience a range of very difficult and ongoing physical and psychological symptoms that are commonly minimized or misunderstood by those untrained and unfamiliar with them (Kazdin et al., 2017; Treasure et al., 2020; Tse et al., 2022). Effective and accessible treatment is of paramount importance given that EDs are associated with elevated mortality risk, physical health complications, and widespread psychological distress and impairment; they can severely decrease quality of life (Arcelus et al., 2011; Mitchison & Hay, 2014).

At the time of this writing, the *Diagnostic and Statistical Manual of Mental Disorders* (DSM-5-TR; American Psychiatric Association, 2022) identifies seven distinct EDs: anorexia nervosa (AN), bulimia nervosa (BN), binge-eating disorder (BED), avoidant–restrictive food intake disorder (ARFID), rumination syndrome, pica, and other specified feeding/eating disorder (OSFED). Though unique in some ways, each of the seven defined EDs shares three key features:

1. They are all characterized by the inability to adequately feed oneself (whether due to fears of the body changing, sensory difficulties, fears of aversive consequences, or problems with appetite-regulating hormones).
2. They are rooted in biological and neurometabolic processes (and not socially constructed illnesses, choices, or dieting fads).

3. They are associated with unique and pervasive psychological features (e.g., anxiety, emotional regulation difficulties, perfectionism) that distinguish them from disordered eating.

Definitions and diagnosis of EDs continue to evolve alongside new research findings. It is important for those in the field to stay current with respect to challenges and concerns with the diagnostic criteria—for example, use of BMI (body mass index) to differentiate between AN and BN; use of the term "atypical" anorexia; or controversy over whether ARFID does or does not involve body image disturbance (Thomas et al., 2023; Herpertz-Dahlmann, 2021; Sharpe, 2024).

## Traditional/Frontline ED Treatments: A Brief Overview

EDs have long posed significant challenges in the fields of psychiatry and psychology. Historically, the treatment of EDs was often inconsistent and rudimentary, largely because these conditions were poorly understood. In the early to mid-20th century, psychoanalytic approaches predominated, focusing on underlying psychological conflicts. However, these methods often lacked empirical support, and many patients continued to struggle with their symptoms despite long-term therapy. The 1970s and 1980s marked a significant shift with the emergence of cognitive-behavioral therapy (CBT) and family-based treatment (FBT), each playing a crucial role in the management of different aspects and stages of these complex conditions (Fairburn et al., 1995; Lock et al., 2010).

CBT-ED, or CBT adapted for EDs, has become the most widely studied and utilized treatment for BN and BED, with robust evidence supporting its effectiveness (Wilson et al., 2007). CBT-ED is a broad term that encompasses several types of cognitive behavioral interventions for individuals suffering from an ED and is grounded in the theory that dysfunctional thoughts and behaviors surrounding food, body image, and self-worth are central to the maintenance of the disorder (Fairburn, 2008; Fairburn, Marcus, & Wilson, 1993). CBT-ED treatments typically involve 20 sessions over 5 months, where patients work to identify and challenge problematic cognitions related to eating, develop stable and regular eating patterns, and learn coping strategies. Numerous studies have demonstrated the efficacy of CBT interventions, reporting significant reductions in binge eating and purging behaviors, as well as improvements in associated psychological symptoms such as depression and anxiety (Murphy et al., 2010; Linardon et al., 2017). For example, a landmark study by Fairburn et al. (1993) found that CBT-ED was superior to interpersonal therapy (IPT) and behavior therapy (BT) in reducing bulimic symptoms at a 1-year follow-up. More recent research has also explored the application of CBT-ED in treating anorexia nervosa, though the evidence suggests it is less effective as a standalone treatment for this population, particularly in severe cases (Treasure & Schmidt, 2013). For clarification: throughout this book we reference CBT-ED as well as CBT-E (enhanced cognitive behavior therapy). As stated above, we use the term CBT-ED to refer to a broad range of cognitive behavioral treatments specifically designed to treat EDs. CBT-E (Fairburn, 2008) is a unique CBT-ED that has been widely studied and shown to be effective in the treatment of AN, BN, and BED.

Family-based treatment (FBT), also known as the Maudsley approach, has emerged as a first-line approach for adolescents with AN, emphasizing the critical role of family support in recovery (Lock & Le Grange, 2013). Developed at the Maudsley Hospital in London in the 1970s, FBT involves the entire family in the treatment process, empowering parents to take an active role in restoring their child's weight and normalizing eating behaviors. FBT is typically conducted over 20 sessions across three phases: (1) weight restoration, where parents are supported in refeeding their child; (2) returning control over eating back to the adolescent; and (3) addressing broader family and adolescent issues to support the maintenance of recovery. The effectiveness of FBT has been supported by several randomized controlled trials (RCTs). For instance, a study by Lock et al. (2010) found that FBT was more effective than adolescent-focused therapy (AFT) in achieving full remission of anorexia nervosa symptoms at a 1-year follow-up. The benefits of FBT are particularly pronounced in younger patients and those with a shorter duration of illness, with evidence suggesting that early intervention with FBT can lead to long-lasting recovery (Couturier et al., 2013; Doyle & Le Grange 2019; Madden et al., 2015).

While traditional treatments like CBT and FBT have laid a strong empirical foundation and remain essential components of eating disorder care, they do not sufficiently address the needs of all individuals. In particular, clients with high emotional reactivity, chronic dysregulation, or comorbid conditions often require a more nuanced and flexible approach—one that explicitly targets the emotional and behavioral complexities often seen in those for whom standard approaches are not adequate. Dialectical behavior therapy (DBT) emerged as a compelling candidate to fill this gap.

## DBT and Eating Disorders

### What Is DBT?

DBT is a sophisticated and integrative therapeutic approach that addresses the nuanced interplay between acceptance and change in individuals with severe emotional and behavioral dysregulation (Linehan, 1993). DBT is a staged treatment that was developed by Marsha Linehan in the late 1980s to treat individuals with recurrent suicidal and self-injurious behaviors, particularly those with borderline personality disorder (BPD). Principle-driven rather than protocol-driven, DBT relies on specific philosophical and theoretical perspectives. The treatment is grounded in dialectical philosophy, which posits that reality is composed of opposing forces and that change occurs through the synthesis of these opposites, rather than by efforts to find the "right" answer or to eliminate what doesn't fit (Linehan, 1993).

In the therapeutic context, dialectics permeates conceptualization and treatment decisions and is embodied in the ongoing balance between accepting the individual's current experiences with the need for behavioral change to improve well-being. By combining cognitive-behavioral strategies with mindfulness and dialectical principles, DBT provides a powerful framework for helping individuals build a life worth living, marked by emotional balance, effective relationships, and a greater sense of inner peace. While most people initially think of the DBT skills as the hallmark feature of the treatment, DBT's application of stylistic, dialectical, and reciprocal strategies truly differentiate it from other treatment paradigms.

It is also important to highlight that DBT is structured into a series of stages that guide the therapeutic process, addressing different levels of dysfunction and helping individuals progress toward a life worth living. These stages are designed to systematically reduce life-threatening behaviors, improve emotional regulation, enhance quality of life, and ultimately help clients achieve goals aligned with their values. Briefly, Stage 1 focuses on achieving behavioral control and reducing life-threatening and severe behavioral issues. Stage 2 addresses past traumas and reduces ongoing emotional pain that tends to reignite Stage 1 behaviors. Stage 3 shifts the focus to improving the quality of everyday life and achieving longer-term personal goals. Stage 4 involves finding a sense of completeness or a deeper sense of meaning and purpose in life. This staged approach allows for a structured and systematic path to recovery, guiding individuals from managing severe behavioral issues to achieving emotional stability and eventually building a

**TABLE 1.1 The Stages of DBT**

| Stage | Challenge | Goal |
|---|---|---|
| Stage 1 | Severe behavioral dyscontrol | Establishing stability |
| Stage 2 | Quiet misery | Emotional processing and experiencing |
| Stage 3 | Problems in living | Navigating ordinary happiness and unhappiness |
| Stage 4 | Incompleteness | Capacity for sustained joy |

fulfilling, meaningful life. Each stage builds upon the last, with the ultimate goal of helping clients not just survive but thrive, by equipping them with the skills and insights needed to lead a balanced and purposeful life (Table 1.1).

## Our Personal Path to DBT

DBT caught our attention because of the translational nature of the work to the clients we wanted to treat—patients who do not respond adequately to standard ED care or whose presentations worsened in the context of those models (Touyz et al., 2023). DBT has been extensively researched and is widely recognized for its effectiveness in reducing self-harm, suicidal behaviors, emotional dysregulation, and the need for emergency services or high levels of care (Kliem et al., 2010). Given that so many of our patients struggle with these same symptoms and patterns, utilizing DBT made a lot of sense to us. Given the widespread success of DBT to treat a condition once considered treatment resistant (i.e., BPD), DBT has evolved into a versatile therapeutic approach that is applied to a wide range of psychological conditions characterized by emotional dysregulation, including eating disorders, substance use disorders, and posttraumatic stress disorder (PTSD) (Antuña-Camblor et al., 2024; Lungu & Linehan, 2016). Full DBT treatment, which we reference throughout this book, involves individual DBT therapy, group skills training, phone coaching, and a consultation team meeting for therapists.

## The Early Days of MED-DBT

The first significant adaptations of DBT for eating disorders began in the mid-1990s and early 2000s, as clinicians and researchers recognized the overlap between the emotional dysregulation seen in BPD and the patterns of impulsive behavior and emotional distress common in eating disorders. During this period, small-scale studies and case reports began to emerge focused on modified DBT skills training for bulimia (DBT-BN) and binge-eating disorder (DBT-BED), also referred to as the Stanford model (Safer et al., 2001a and b, 2009). This approach continues to be utilized and studied in patients with BN or BED (Safer et al., 2017; Rahmani et al., 2018) and has been adapted to include a guided self-help option that has been shown to be effective for patients with BED (Masson et al., 2013; Carter, Kennedy, Singleton, Van Wijk, & Heath, 2019).

While we were both interested in this work, we recognized that these frameworks were not designed for the people we wanted to help. The Stanford model and the guided self-help protocol were intended for individuals with primary EDs in the mild to moderate range and focused predominantly on teaching DBT skills in a group or one-on-one context. We view DBT skills as essential, but we believe that those with multidiagnostic presentations require the full DBT framework to maximize success. The dialectical stance, target hierarchy, DBT assumptions, focus on emotional and interpersonal regulation, and the application of DBT skills were highly beneficial, but our clients simultaneously needed help with eating, developing a different relationship with food, managing weight and medical stability, and navigating body image distress.

The model that we have developed draws heavily from the CBT for ED treatment literature, and there is much that is consistent with the CBT for ED model within DBT. That being said, there are many differences between the two models. It has been our personal and professional experience that clinicians who are expertly trained in DBT have no trouble managing suicidality, self-injury, and therapy-interfering behaviors (TIBs), but are prone to fear and avoidance when it comes to weighing their clients, prescribing that they eat three meals and two snacks per day, managing medical instability, or integrating food and fluid intake as part of a diary card. On the other hand, ED therapists are comfortable with the ins and outs of psychoeducation around EDs, managing medical concerns secondary to EDs, and are experts at evaluating a food log but become fearful and avoidant when their client expresses suicidality, engages in self-injurious behaviors, or may ask the client to leave treatment if they engage in therapy-interfering behaviors such as water loading or refusing to eat.

Our work was bolstered by several other studies at that time that demonstrated promise in the adapted use of DBT for patients with multidiagnostic EDs. Results from case series designs showed feasibility, acceptability, reductions in purging behaviors and binge eating, and improvements in mood, emotion regulation, and treatment retention among those who had not responded to frontline ED approaches (Ben-Porath et al., 2009; Chen et al., 2008; Kröger et al., 2010; Palmer et al., 2003; Salbach-Andrae et al., 2008; see review by Bankoff et al., 2012).

Together, we delivered, refined, and evaluated the MED-DBT protocol in both adult (Federici et al., 2012; Federici & Wisniewski, 2013) and adolescent (Federici & Wisniewski, 2012) populations. We spent a great deal of time reading, consulting, and discussing alternative treatment models, including specialist supportive clinical management (SSCM) and radically open DBT (RO-DBT). While both contained elements that were helpful (e.g., a focus on quality of life, targeting rigidity and social signaling), these protocols were still not sufficient for the needs of our patients. The program we implemented and evaluated entailed a minimum commitment to 6 months of MED-DBT where patients attended either day treatment programming (6 hours/day, 5 days/week) or intensive outpatient programming (IOP; 3 hours/day, 3–5 days/week). Predominantly group-based, patients attend weekly individual DBT therapy, regular nutrition and psychiatry appointments, and have access to between-session skills coaching.

The case series we published in 2013 followed seven women with longstanding and multidiagnostic EDs over 6 months (Federici & Wisniewski, 2013). Treatment completion for all of the patients was associated with reductions in ED symptoms, suicidal and self-injurious behaviors, therapy-interfering behaviors, psychiatric and medical hospitalizations, and clinician burnout (Federici & Wisniewski, 2013). The feedback we received from patients and staff was inspiring and we were motivated by the manner in which the model reinvigorated treatment for people who felt little else could be done for them. We continued to explore how the model impacted affect regulation (Ben-Porath et al., 2014), what skills were more impactful at meals (Marek et al., 2013), and how to utilize contingency management protocols and establishing novel dialectical dilemmas specific to our patients (Wisniewski & Ben-Porath, 2015).

## What about RO-DBT?

An alternative framework, RO-DBT (radically open DBT), has emerged as a possible treatment pathway for patients with anorexia who present as emotionally overcontrolled. Certainly, across ED diagnoses, some patients struggle with low novelty-seeking (Rossier et al., 2000), heightened threat sensitivity (Harrison, Sullivan, Tchanturia, & Treasure, 2010), low sensitivity to reward (Harrison, O'Brien, Lopez, & Treasure, 2010), cognitive rigidity (Tchanturia et al., 2012), inhibited emotional expression/recognition (Geller, Cockell, Hewitt, Goldner, & Flett, 2000), and loneliness (Zucker et al., 2007). RO-DBT theorizes that these bio-temperamental characteristics cause and maintain ED behaviors (Hemple et al., 2018). This specific theory of overcontrol as it applies to restrictive ED behaviors has yet to be empirically tested; however, several studies have been published showing promising outcomes including a case study (Little & Codd, 2020); an open, uncontrolled trial of 47 patients on an inpatient ED unit (Lynch et al., 2013), a qualitative analysis (Isaksson et al., 2021); an uncontrolled study of 131 adolescents in a day treatment setting in which RO-DBT groups were embedded (Baudinet et al., 2020); and an outpatient feasibility study of 23 patients with AN (Ejdemyr et al, 2025).

While promising, these studies have excluded patients with low body weights, those with binge/purge behaviors, cognitive difficulties, BPD symptoms and, in some cases, patients needing more intensive ED support or those who had recently participated in other treatments. In the two larger studies commonly cited to support the use of RO-DBT for anorexia nervosa restricting type (AN-R), patients were concurrently involved in high levels of ED care where weight, eating, and other ED interventions were employed. Given the lack of a waitlist control group or randomized controlled trial, it is difficult to determine whether the observed improvements are due to the passage of time, more traditional ED interventions, nonspecific effects of general inpatient or outpatient treatment, or the specific impact of RO-DBT (Ben-Porath et al., 2020).

In our own training/consultation with the RO-DBT treatment developers, we struggled to make it work for our clients. It is our view that RO-DBT may be a useful treatment for some patients as a Stage 3 treatment but not as a Stage 1 or 2 model (see Thomas et al., 2024). Our clients require intensive support to stay alive, including maintaining medical stability alongside reducing suicidal and self-injurious behaviors. They need help reducing the behaviors that get in the way of participating in treatment, including cognitive challenges secondary to food restriction and weight loss. They require a model that can help them manage emotions (including fear, disgust, and envy), especially around food, meal planning, and navigating weight gain or other bodily sensations that are distressing. Moreover, we have found that emotional overcontrol and undercontrol tendencies coexist in our patients. We are not convinced that these are binary constructs, rather that our patients can and do experience both. For example, our clients can present as highly overcontrolled until they have to eat or gain weight.

## Summary

Over the past 15 years, we have seen an increase in the number of published studies showing that MED-DBT reduces both ED and BPD symptoms and increases treatment engagement across levels of care including outpatient (Courbasson et al., 2012; Liakopoulou et al., 2023; Navarro-Haro et al., 2018), day treatment (Brown et al., 2018; McColl, Donkin, & Hindle, 2024; Pennell et al., 2019), and partial hospitalization (Brown et al., 2019a, 2019b). Several research groups are currently working on more robust clinical trials for MED-DBT, and it will be important to continue to modify or adapt our model based on the evolving literature. The information in this chapter will be important for you to share with your client as needed and to weave into early discussions about why they might consider MED-DBT compared to other available models. In the following chapter, we walk you through our criteria for MED-DBT and recommendations for assessing suitability.

# 2

# Assessment for Treatment

## Is MED-DBT a Good Fit for Your Client?

Assessing your client is essential to determine whether MED-DBT is appropriate or whether another treatment approach would be indicated. In order to do this, you need to know if your client has an ED, the level of symptom severity if so, and how the ED fits into the context of their co-occurring diagnoses. We spend a significant amount of time making sure that DBT is the treatment recommendation before moving forward. Once we know that DBT is the appropriate treatment, we need to determine *which* type of DBT to recommend (e.g., standard DBT, MED-DBT, DBT-BN). This last determination is influenced by the co-occurring difficulties your client struggles with as well as the other treatments they have already tried. Once we have decided that DBT is the recommended treatment for this particular individual, and we have ascertained that MED-DBT is recommended, only then can we move to the pretreatment motivation and commitment phase.

### Determining the Treatment Pathway

Over the years, we have developed a set of criteria to determine whether a trial of MED-DBT might be indicated. We recommend that you consider offering MED-DBT if the client with an ED has experienced two or more of the following:

- Unsuccessful attempts with outpatient evidence-based ED treatment (e.g., CBT-ED, FBT, IPT) and/or unsuccessful attempts in higher levels of care
- Recurrent suicidal or self-injurious behavior

- Persistent emotion regulation difficulties and/or reports that the ED functions as a way to manage emotions
- History of therapy-interfering behaviors

It is also important to clarify and confirm with your client that they have, in fact, received an adequate dose of an evidence-based ED treatment. Many clients will report to us that they have tried FBT or CBT-ED; however, on further exploration we learn that they have not received or been exposed to food monitoring, collaborative weights, or typical homework assignments around eating, weight, and body image.

In addition to assessing for an ED and the level of severity, we recommend assessing for the following symptoms, as these are the most common comorbidities:

- Emotion regulation
- BPD
- Depression
- Anxiety
- Trauma
- OCD
- Substance use disorders

This can be accomplished via questionnaires, semi-structured interviews, or both. For a more comprehensive guide on assessing EDs, refer to Waller et al. (2007) and Fairburn (2008).

## Case Studies

For some clients, the assessment will provide clear direction and MED-DBT will be an obvious choice (e.g., the client meets many of the eligibility criteria), while for others, the treatment recommendation may be less clear. You may find yourself wondering which evidence-based treatment (EBT) to offer your client. We will describe three cases to highlight how to think through your treatment recommendations.

### Case 1: Kelly

Kelly is a 46-year-old married woman who has struggled with BED since she was 18 years old. She is a full-time administrative coordinator at a busy law firm and a mom to two children. She described eating three meals per day, "grazing" on snacks between meals, and binge eating most evenings. She said she feels out of control during binges. Since she often doesn't know when she is full, she eats until she feels really uncomfortable. She reported trying many diets over the past 25 years, which resulted in weight cycling. She said she is ashamed of her body and her "lack of willpower over eating." Kelly described problems managing emotions and noted that binge episodes are often the result of feeling shame, anxiety, or sadness. She is embarrassed to eat with others and has limited social interactions outside of work. She said she doesn't really understand her feelings and was always taught to suppress or hide them. She recalled a few times as a teenager when she thought she would "be better off dead" when she was bullied for her weight and shape; however, Kelly denied any thoughts of suicide since that time and has no history of self-injury. Kelly attended an outpatient CBT group for BED in the past and went to an ED psychoeducation course offered at the local hospital a few years ago but said these haven't led to any lasting changes. She says her goals for treatment are to "better manage my emotions" and feel less "out of control with eating."

### Case 2: Jackie

Jackie is a 21-year-old cisgender woman who developed AN when she was 12 years old. At the age of 14, she was sexually assaulted at a middle school graduation party, which caused persistent PTSD. Unable to manage the ED and trauma, Jackie reported intense urges to kill herself, which her parents struggled to manage. Jackie said she still has a desire to die and cuts her thighs and arms at least once per week. She has had three near-lethal suicide attempts, one at age 15, another at 19, and one a couple of months ago. She uses cannabis most days and has a recent history of alcohol and cocaine abuse. She is at a low body weight and reported that the low weight helps to reduce urges for suicide and self-injury. She restricts her eating most days, is highly active, and purges once/week. She was treated with FBT, interspersed with numerous hospitalizations between the ages of 12 and 17. When she turned 18, she moved out of her parent's house to live with her girlfriend, subsequently losing more weight. Soon after, she was admitted to an adult inpatient ED unit due to bradycardia and chest pains. Since then, Jackie has been in and out of day treatment and inpatient programs and attempted outpatient therapy with different providers mainly applying CBT-ED or supportive treatments. She tried eye movement desensitization and reprocessing (EMDR) at age 20 and CPT at age 18 to address trauma but this increased suicidal urges, self-injury, and restriction which led to acute medical instability. Jackie struggles to navigate boundaries and emotions which has made previous treatment experiences difficult as she often forms intense and inappropriate bonds with co-patients or healthcare providers. As you do your assessment, she tells you that she doubts anyone can help her and that she doesn't know if she wants to even try more treatment at this time.

### Case 3: Ryan

Ryan is a 28-year-old transgender male who lives alone. He has struggled with body image issues and "atypical" anorexia since age 15. He only recently disclosed his symptoms and has never received treatment for the ED. When a friend encouraged him to talk with his doctor about his symptoms, he reported that the doctor dismissed his concerns and said his weight was "just fine" and that "people with eating disorders are at much lower weights." Ryan had started to punch himself and pinch his skin when he was in his late teens and noted that he occasionally engages in these behaviors when he feels overwhelmed. He has occasional thoughts of ending his life but has never made an attempt. He struggles with his emotions, reports not understanding what he is feeling much of the time, and tends to cope by suppressing, masking, and being highly perfectionistic. Ryan has cycled through periods of restriction and weight loss and periods of binge eating and purging. He suffers from concentration problems, heart palpitations, cold intolerance, and hair loss. He feels incredibly uncomfortable in his skin and does not want to work on anything that might increase body weight. He described a substantial history of invalidation including bullying, emotional neglect, and physical assault. He is very wary about engaging in ED treatment because he worries that people will not understand his experience as a transgender male or as someone with "atypical" anorexia. When you explain treatment options and recommend a trial of CBT-ED first, Ryan does not want to participate in that model and prefers to start right away with MED-DBT.

## Which DBT to Use?

Given what we know about DBT and its focus on multiple problems, life-threatening symptoms, emotion regulation, and invalidating environments, we might consider using DBT to help Kelly, Jackie, and Ryan. But *which* DBT is right for these individuals?

As we highlighted in Chapter 1, individuals with primary ED presentations (not multidiagnostic) in the mild to moderate severity range, and who would be conceptualized as being in Stage 3, may be well-suited for DBT-BED or DBT-BN (i.e., the Stanford model). This model would be appropriate for a case like Kelly's. For Jackie, given her suicidal ideation (SI) and self-harm (SH), trauma history, and pervasive emotional and interpersonal dysregulation, the Stanford model would not be sufficient. For Ryan, the sole focus on skills training would be inadequate to help with issues of trust, interpersonal regulation, coping with invalidation, and addressing ambivalence about targeting the ED. In addition, as skills-only interventions, DBT-BED and DBT-BN are silent on the intersection between EDs, gender, sexual orientation, and the unique ways people in the 2SLGBTQ+ community have been invalidated, which would be essential to your work with Ryan.

Radically open DBT was developed as a treatment for people struggling with emotional overcontrol characterized by excessively rigid thinking patterns, social isolation, an aloof and distant style of communication, and difficulty with social signaling. While Ryan displays some of these characteristics, RO-DBT was not designed as a Stage 1 treatment for EDs and does not integrate ED psychoeducation, medical and nutritional monitoring, navigate body image disturbances, or adapt diary cards to help with feeding and eating. In our experience, RO-DBT may be a useful intervention for clients in Stage 3 but does not provide the structure or support for clients who actively need help with weight and nutritional stability, life-threatening ED behaviors, and emotional and interpersonal regulation. Kelly, Jackie, and Ryan are all in Stage 1 and require help with both eating and body image in addition to emotion regulation.

## What If My Client Wants to Start with MED-DBT?

Ryan has not tried one of the standard ED evidence-based treatments and stated that he did not wish to engage in a trial of CBT-E or IPT. He requested starting with MED-DBT because he read about it and the approach resonated with him. Can a client bypass standard ED treatments?

Given research evidence supporting CBT and FBT, we generally recommend that clients try these modalities first before attempting a trial of MED-DBT. These models have more empirical support and are generally less expensive. This is usually not an issue because our clients typically have histories of several unsuccessful treatment attempts by the time they are being assessed for MED-DBT. That said, for clients like Ryan who may not have had access to one of the EBTs and/or those who want to begin in MED-DBT, it is important to review the pros and cons of starting with MED-DBT. The patient's views must be considered when determining the treatment pathway. We would recommend talking with Ryan to ensure he has a solid understanding of what CBT-ED involves and highlight that there is more research support for CBT at this time. It would be necessary for him to gain an understanding of the research and the important theoretical differences between MED-DBT and CBT. A discussion about the fact that MED-DBT has a greater time and financial commitment compared to CBT-ED would also be indicated. In this case, Ryan felt that the focus on emotions and managing pervasive invalidation coupled with the multimodal nature of MED-DBT was a better fit for him.

## Would a Trial of Standard DBT (without the Focus on ED) Be Helpful First?

Jackie presents with multiple areas of difficulty including emotional dysregulation, interpersonal ups and downs, impulsivity, suicide, and self-injury. In addition to the ED, she suffers from PTSD and has significant ambivalence about recovery and treatment. If she continues to cycle in and out of treatments that were not designed for her, Jackie is likely to become more entrenched in unhelpful behaviors. Standard ED approaches have not helped. Skills-only approaches are not enough. RO-DBT is not organized to address all of Jackie's medical, nutritional, and psychological needs.

Given Jackie's symptoms, some clinicians might suggest a trial of standard DBT for her. However, we have found that, while DBT-trained clinicians are comfortable and effective in targeting suicide and self-injury and TIBs, they lack training and expertise in targeting ED behaviors such as providing ED psychoeducation, weighing clients, monitoring food and fluid intake, helping with body image distress, and determining when and how to collaborate with a medical provider around the ED. In fact, given our combined experience training DBT therapists in the MED-DBT model, many DBT therapists are uncomfortable or afraid to talk about weight, food, and eating with their clients. When clients like Jackie participate in standard DBT, they feel validated, value the skills, and may see a reduction in suicide and self-injury—and the ED often remains intact even after 1 year of treatment. Therefore, with a framework for managing both the ED and the emotion regulation difficulties, MED-DBT may be the most viable care pathway for Jackie.

It has been encouraging to see more ED services include DBT skills training in their program offerings (e.g., IOP, day treatment). Like

DBT-BED and DBT-BN, this could be another option for Kelly, who would have more support around symptom interruption while learning skills to manage emotions and distress. We have found that clients like Jackie, and likely Ryan, need more than an environment that just adds DBT skills to a predominantly FBT or CBT-ED focused setting since these programs often do not embody the DBT treatment assumptions, team agreements, and do not offer the multimodal functions that MED-DBT provides. Clients like Jackie and Ryan tend to do better in environments that apply dialectical theory, use DBT protocols for managing TIBs, use the target hierarchy, focus on secondary targets, and apply DBT commitment strategies.

## Levels of Severity and MED-DBT

As you assess clients, the severity of the ED and a determination regarding the level of care (LOC) is necessary. Published guidelines (Academy for Eating Disorders, 2023) recommend more intensive support (e.g., day treatment, residential, inpatient) when clients are:

- Rapidly deteriorating medically or psychiatrically
- Presenting with acute medical risk
- Showing suicidality
- Suffering from co-occurring symptoms that interfere with outpatient treatment (e.g., substance use, difficulty managing anger)
- Experiencing daily symptoms that interfere with the quality of life
- Not ready to change, display poor insight, and/or do not have psychosocial support to manage feeding or safety concerns outside of the hospital setting (APA, 2023)

These recommendations make sense in the absence of a viable outpatient model that can manage the needs of our clients. These guidelines also make sense when a client has not yet tried them. Given that CBT, IPT, and FBT are not equipped to handle EDs in the context of comorbid conditions, multiple high-risk behaviors, and behaviors that interfere with treatment, higher LOCs (HLOC) would be a natural next step. However, once a client has attempted the higher levels of care without long-term success, the advantages of using these approaches are unclear and could reinforce passivity and the sick role.

The model we have developed, however, has been built to help people who struggle with an ED in the context of other co-occurring conditions *in an outpatient model of care*. Therefore, your assessment helps you to determine whether your client's symptoms, including suicide and medical risk, can be managed in the context of MED-DBT and whether you have the experience, training, and support to provide the treatment.

These are tough decisions. Given clients' ambivalence and multiple high-risk behaviors, it makes sense that many clinicians are uncomfortable treating our clients on an outpatient basis. It is our experience that these clients are often too quickly referred to day treatment or inpatient settings. This is similar to the way BPD was managed before DBT was developed. Patients with recurrent suicidal and self-injurious behaviors were commonly admitted (and readmitted) to inpatient units for months, sometimes years. While this provided a degree of comfort to patients, families, and/or health practitioners, it did not treat the condition. In fact, research has shown that repeated hospitalizations for suicide/self-injury in adult and adolescent populations have unintended negative effects including an increased risk of completed suicide (Czyz et al., 2016; Goldman-Mellor et al., 2022). We have to keep in mind that DBT (as an outpatient model) was designed (and is effective) for severe and high-risk individuals who have not responded to traditional approaches (usually incorrectly deemed "treatment resistant") struggling with emotional and interpersonal dysregulation.

How does this relate to the assessment of our clients? Although HLOC are recommended for suicide, co-occurring psychiatric illnesses, and ambivalence in those with EDs, they predominantly rely on CBT or FBT principles and are managed through the lens of the medical model. While essential (in many cases) for saving lives through the provision of feeding and medical stability, these approaches can have negative effects on clients. After all, these are the same models that did not work in the outpatient setting. The question is, do repeated hospitalizations for ED severity in our client population lead to meaningful change? Maybe, for some. For many, however, engaging in a treatment model that was not designed to meet their needs can inadvertently be experienced as invalidating, traumatizing, and can exacerbate symptoms. While more day treatment and residential ED programs are including DBT skills in their programs, this is not the same as providing comprehensive MED-DBT. As a result, most settings do not administer therapy models designed for severe emotional and interpersonal dysregulation, personality disorders, suicide and self-injury, or persistent ambivalence alongside ED treatment, even though clients are being referred to HLOC for those reasons.

As MED-DBT providers, we must assess the dialectical tension between the medical and safety needs of our clients with the knowledge that this could be managed in MED-DBT and that most of our clients are not well served/helped in standard HLOC programs. Keep in mind as well that MED-DBT is a more intensive treatment than other outpatient models (e.g., 3+ hours per week plus 24/7 phone coaching vs. 1–2 hours in standard outpatient models) and is designed to manage chronic ED presentations. So, you are assessing whether there is a level of acuteness that cannot be managed in pretreatment: in the full model that would be better suited by a day treatment or inpatient setting.

First and foremost, the determination of LOC rests on knowing your personal/professional limits as well as the limits of the system in which you and your clients exist. If you are in an environment without a team and without ED and DBT expertise, we recommend that you follow the American Psychiatric Association guidelines (2023). If, however, you are a clinician with expertise managing multidiagnostic and high-risk clients, and have a team, you may consider using this model in lieu of a HLOC.

## Summary

Therapists in MED-DBT need support, and decisions about severity and treatment recommendations need the help of the MED-DBT-trained team. The assessment is the initial step in determining whether MED-DBT is the right approach for a particular client. You will need to know if there is an ED present and how that relates to their co-occurring conditions and their treatment history. If you decide that a DBT model is the treatment of choice, you then need to figure out *which* DBT to use. Once the determination is made that MED-DBT is the appropriate treatment choice, your client can begin the MED-DBT pretreatment phase.

Determining whether a client is a good fit for MED-DBT involves more than assessing symptom severity or diagnostic categories—it requires a shared understanding of why previous treatments may have fallen short and what makes this approach different. To that end, a strong therapeutic alliance begins not only with validation but also with a compelling and personalized theory that helps clients make sense of their suffering and that gives them hope for change.

In the next chapter, we introduce the biosocial theory that underpins MED-DBT and explore how it shapes every aspect of the treatment—from case conceptualization to intervention.

# PART II

# MED-DBT Theories and Treatment Assumptions

This part of the book provides information on the theories that will guide your clinical conceptualizations and direct treatment decisions (e.g., the adapted biosocial theory, dialectical dilemmas, MED-DBT treatment assumptions), alongside a description of how to build your MED-DBT team. Deciding to work in this model requires agreement on why our clients struggle and why other treatments may have been less effective. The MED-DBT team agrees ahead of time to approach their clinical work within the theories, principles, and assumptions described in this section of the text. Likewise, a solid understanding of these treatment elements is necessary as you will need to explain them to your clients in the pretreatment phase.

This part of the book includes the following:

- Chapter 3: Introduction to the Adapted Biosocial Theory: A Focus on Biology
- Chapter 4: The Adapted Biosocial Theory: A Focus on Invalidating Environments
- Chapter 5: Assumptions about MED-DBT Clients
- Chapter 6: Building Your MED-DBT Team
- Chapter 7: Dialectical Dilemmas in MED-DBT Treatment

# 3

# Introduction to the Adapted Biosocial Theory

## A Focus on Biology

If you are using an evidence-based treatment, the theories you use to understand how symptoms arise and are maintained govern the entire treatment process; they direct assessment practices, moment-by-moment interactions, treatment structure, treatment planning, and how we, as therapists, respond to our client's behaviors in and out of session.

Each psychological treatment has its own set of theories and proposed mechanisms of change. For example, CBT-ED theorizes that eating disorders develop and persist due to problematic ways of thinking about food, weight, and body shape (Fairburn, 2008). CBT models for EDs therefore focus on modifying cognition through psychoeducation, tracking food and weight, challenging ED beliefs and assumptions, and through the use of food and body-based exposure exercises. FBT, another evidence-based treatment for adolescents with EDs, is agnostic regarding the development of the ED and does not seek an explanation for it (Lock & LeGrange, 2013). The mechanisms of change in FBT include parental empowerment and utilizing the family system to provide nourishment and stabilization.

These theories and treatment approaches, while incredibly helpful for many, do not apply to all individuals with EDs. In fact, many clients who have not responded adequately to standard evidence-based treatments report feeling that the treatment philosophies were a poor fit and/or that the approaches were insufficient in explaining and reducing their difficulties (Downs, 2024a and b; Federici & Wisniewski, 2015; Reay, Holliday, Stewart, & Adams, 2022; Wisniewski, Safer, & Chen, 2007; Vinchenzo, Lawrence, & McCombie, 2022). Not surprisingly, this can have a profoundly negative impact on those who have cycled in and out of standard ED approaches. Given that approximately 50% of patients are not adequately helped by standard approaches, many clients have internalized a deep sense of hopelessness (Downs et al., 2023). Studies have shown that when treatments fail our clients, preexisting beliefs or fears of being too complex, misunderstood, and abandoned are exacerbated (Johns et al., 2019; Vinchenzo et al., 2022). By the time most clients reach our MED-DBT services, there is a palpable sense of dejection, mistrust, and/or exhaustion in thinking about trying yet another therapy model.

While DBT utilizes standard cognitive and behavioral interventions, the theory regarding how problems arise and are maintained is fundamentally different. DBT is an *emotion*-based treatment that theorizes that symptoms develop due to biological differences in self-regulation in the context of chronic invalidation (Niedtfeld & Bohus, 2018). While more research is needed to clarify whether all people with EDs exhibit these conditions, the application of DBT to EDs allows for both cognitive and emotional conceptualizations, rather than just the cognitive. Thus, in order to generate hope and regenerate interest in trying a new treatment, the therapist first engages the client in a collaborative discussion about the MED-DBT approach, focusing on the adapted biosocial theory. A shared understanding of how the ED developed alongside other disorders, why it is maintained, and why other treatments may not have been effective is essential.

Moreover, MED-DBT creates space for clients to learn how to address their co-occurring symptoms as well as to learn to simultaneously think about and cope with the number of problems that many people who have EDs face. Clients are much more likely to engage with treatment when they feel understood, their experiences are validated, and when the treatment itself makes sense and provides a way to move forward. Treatment success depends on a strong and compassionate formulation of the individual's problems. Helping clients understand that they and their problems make sense is imperative to the model.

This chapter focuses on the critical biological and neurodevelopmental factors that must be added to the original biosocial theory to fully account for ED symptomatology. Chapter 4 then explores how chronic invalidation interacts with these vulnerabilities to shape the client's trajectory and influence treatment needs. This model is designed to be shared in a highly collaborative and exploratory manner in which you and your client evaluate and discuss these concepts with respect to whether and how they apply to their life experiences. The adaptations to the biosocial theory assume you are well-versed in current ED knowledge, including diagnostic features, causes (e.g., genetics, metabolic, sociocultural factors), weight science, weight stigma, medical and psychological complications, risk assessment, as well as the nondieting approaches to stabilizing eating.

# The Original Biosocial Theory

The original biosocial theory was developed as a way to explain how borderline personality disorder (BPD) develops (Linehan, 1993). The theory describes a unique transactional relationship between an emotionally sensitive person and a chronically invalidating environment. The biological underpinnings of BPD are thought to originate in altered brain regions related to emotion regulation, impulse control, threat sensitivity, and reward system processes (Meyer-Lindenberg et al., 2006; Ochsner & Gross, 2014). We assume the reader is familiar with the biosocial theory, so only a brief review of the model is provided here.

## Linehan's Biosocial Theory for BPD

The "bio" part of the biosocial theory addresses unique genetic factors that predispose people to the development of BPD. Due to proposed differences in the limbic system and additional brain regions associated with impulsivity, threat sensitivity, and reward versus punishment processes, people who develop BPD are biologically "primed" to display the following characteristics (Niedtfeld & Bohus, 2018):

1. *Emotional sensitivity:* A tendency to assign emotional meaning or valence to stimuli, to interpret ambiguous information as emotionally significant, and to exhibit vigilance for possible emotional threat. In essence, the brain is primed to detect threats and to process incoming information as emotional in nature.
2. *Intense emotional experiencing:* Individuals living with BPD have a biological propensity to feel emotions with greater intensity and for longer durations compared to those without BPD.
3. *Slow to return to baseline:* Primed to detect emotions and threat more fluidly and hardwired to experience strong affective states, individuals with BPD take longer to return to emotional baseline once triggered. For example, those without this biology might experience shame or anger but be able to regulate themselves to continue with their work or school obligations, whereas someone with this particular biology will

find it very difficult to re-regulate and may be unable to carry on effectively with their day. When the brain is "wired" in this way, people find themselves moving from threat to threat with very little relief in between.

## Chronic Invalidation

While such brain-based predispositions are thought to be necessary for the development of BPD and other illnesses for which emotion regulation is considered to be a core feature, they are not sufficient on their own. Many people with this particular biotemperament do not go on to develop BPD. Problems with emotions, cognitions, relationships, and behavior are believed to develop when an emotionally sensitive individual is exposed to chronic environmental invalidation. Invalidation is defined as any communication (e.g., verbal or nonverbal) that labels or treats a person's emotions, thoughts, or actions as bad, wrong, unacceptable, nonsensical, and/or unwanted. Invalidating environments can include the family of origin but are usually more wide-reaching than that and can include extended family members, peers, teachers, coaches, and the broader sociocultural context (Fruzzetti, Shenk, & Hoffman, 2005; Linehan, 1993).

As depicted in Figure 3.1 and based on Alan Fruzzetti's work (Fruzzetti, 2006), invalidation exists on a continuum both in terms of intent and severity.

On one side of the continuum, invalidation can occur as a result of being unheard, unseen, or misunderstood in the environment. Often not intentional, the external system may be unaware that there are needs, may misinterpret needs, or may not be able to perceive the world through the eyes of the person suffering. Invalidation at this stage can also occur as fragilization and overprotectiveness, where the dominant communication is that a person is incapable of handling things, coping more effectively, or learning new skills. As you move from left to right on the continuum, the type and intensity of invalidation increases and includes overt bullying,

| **Subtle Invalidation →** | **Persistent Misattunement →** | **Overt/Systemic Harm** |
|---|---|---|
| Ignoring, brushing off, "It's not that bad" | Misreading distress, failed repair, repeated boundary violations | Discrimination, coercion, abuse, systemic harm |

**FIGURE 3.1** The invalidation continuum: From subtle dismissal to overt harm. Copyright © 2026 Anita Federici and Lucene Wisniewski. Reprinted by permission.

marginalization, and oppression. On the far right of the continuum are extreme forms of invalidation, including physical and sexual abuse.

The consequences of repeated invalidation can have a profound impact on anyone, and particularly for those who are emotionally sensitive (Crowell, Beauchaine, & Linehan, 2009). For most people, the experience of being invalidated activates the body's threat system, which mobilizes the emotional center of the brain and prepares the body for possible attack (Greville-Harris, Hempel, Karl, Dieppe, & Lynch, 2016; Shenk & Fruzzetti, 2011). Under these conditions, a person is much less able to absorb new information or respond effectively to others or to the environment. While we all experience some degree of threat activation in the face of invalidation, those who develop BPD have a much harder time moderating the impact as the brain plays a key role in mediating one's capacity to self-regulate and manage invalidation. The combined impact of repeated invalidation in an individual with an emotionally sensitive biology creates a number of unique and problematic outcomes, including the following:

- Deficient self-soothing skills
- Inability to accurately identify emotions
- Poorly regulated emotions/emotional avoidance
- Pervasive self-doubt
- Chronic self-hatred
- Inadequate identity formation
- Poor communication and interpersonal skills
- Black-and-white thinking style
- Discomfort with uncertainty
- Deep sense of emptiness
- Fears of rejection and abandonment
- Reliance on maladaptive coping mechanisms to cope

These profound consequences render a person even more vulnerable to emotions, thus creating a negative feedback loop between biology and environment. The individual is effectively "stuck" in a cycle of extreme emotional sensitivity colliding with invalidation, resulting in pervasive skill deficits leading to more emotional sensitivity and invalidation (Grove & Crowell, 2018).

It is important to highlight that the biosocial theory is nonblaming in nature. The individual is not to blame for being emotionally sensitive: they did not choose their biology. Likewise, the environment on its own is not to blame for causing problems, except in situations of oppression, abuse, or neglect. Rather, problems arise due to the repeated interactions between the environment and the individual (Linehan, 1993).

## Adapting the Biosocial Theory for Multidiagnostic Eating Disorders: A Focus on Biology

The biosocial theory provides a useful framework for understanding many of the difficulties our clients experience; however, adaptations are needed. Eating disorders cannot fully be explained by emotional sensitivity and invalidating environments as currently described by Linehan (1993). Many people with BPD do not have a co-occurring ED, and many people with an ED do not have BPD. To leave the biosocial theory as originally described would give the false impression that EDs are *not* about food and weight and that they can be explained as an emotion regulation disorder. This is not the case. EDs have unique biological and environmental underpinnings that must be taken into account in conceptualization and treatment planning.

For the remainder of this chapter, we focus on biotempermental factors to be added to the biosocial theory. An exploration of the unique invalidating environments that influence our clients follows in Chapter 4.

In the MED-DBT model, it is imperative to adapt the biosocial theory to integrate current genetic and biological markers that drive ED symptomatology. Genetics and neurobiology drive food preferences, weight changes/stability, energy expenditure, digestion, anxiety sensitivity, and body image perception. In order to help patients, the treatment must focus on both the genetics of emotion regulation and that of an ED (Downs, 2024). In our experience, it is not sufficient to target emotions as the primary way to overcome the inability to eat, manage sensory issues related to food and digestion, or treat body image.

With respect to biology, the MED-DBT biosocial theory integrates the following four key areas (though it is important to remember that the biology of EDs is evolving, and it is imperative to stay up-to-date as the science develops and changes):

## Metabolic Differences

Anorexia is increasingly recognized not only as a psychiatric disorder but also as one with profound metabolic underpinnings. Groundbreaking genome-wide association studies (GWAS) led by Bulik and colleagues (Bulik et al., 2019; Bulik et al., 2021; Watson et al., 2019; Duncan et al., 2017) have identified specific genetic loci (or areas on the genome) that have previously been associated with neuropsychiatric, metabolic/anthropometric, and autoimmune traits. In addition, a series of genetic correlations, which measure the extent to which the same genetic variants influence different traits revealed some excepted positive genetic correlations, such as positive genetic correlations between anorexia and OCD, depression, and anxiety, more surprising was a panel of negative genetic correlations with metabolic factors like body mass index (BMI) and type 2 diabetes. What this means is that some of the same genes that increase risk for AN also increase risk for OCD, depression, and anxiety, but some of the same genes that increase risk for AN *decrease* risk for high BMI and type 2 diabetes. This genetic profile has led researchers to recommend that AN be reclassified as a "metabo-psychiatric" condition. These findings also help explain why many individuals with AN relapse shortly after hospital-based weight restoration; the body, in effect, pulls them back down toward an energetically dysregulated state. Biological differences in energy expenditure, pain tolerance, GI function, and hunger/satiety signaling are not just secondary complications of starvation, they may predate the onset of the illness and drive core symptoms in a subset of individuals. Experiences such as early-onset food allergies, dysfunctional [CB1] gastrointestinal functioning, or a heightened sense of reward following caloric restriction all suggest that the biology of AN shapes lived experience.

Recent large-scale genomic work on binge-eating behaviors (Termorshuizen et al., 2025) has further advanced our understanding of EDs by identifying genetic differences *between* ED subtypes. Although psychiatric genetic correlations overlap across EDs, anthropometric genetic correlations diverge significantly: the same genetic factors that increase risk for AN are associated with *lower* risk for obesity, while the genetic factors that increase risk for binge eating are associated with *higher* risk for obesity. These findings further emphasize the importance of integrating metabolic considerations into ED conceptualization and treatment.

As Bulik notes, recovery is often not simply a matter of motivation or willpower, patients are often fighting an uphill battle against their biology. Please see Bulik's article (2024) in which she describes how to explain genetics to patients and families.

## Sensory and Perceptual Differences

EDs are associated with biological differences with respect to body image perception, interoceptive awareness (e.g., the ability to accurately sense and interpret somatic cues), and taste/texture preferences. Research supports that such experiences are "hardwired" and not simply cognitive distortions (Brizzi et al., 2023). For example, individuals with ARFID commonly experience oral sensitivities and hormonal differences that impact the experience of eating, chewing, and swallowing foods (Becker et al., 2021; Burton Murray et al., 2022). From a transdiagnostic perspective, different food textures and smells can be aversive to many who suffer. While disgust sensitivity is linked to an evolutionary adaptation designed to prevent ingestion of toxins and other harmful foods, it may play an important role in those with EDs who find some food types highly aversive. Moreover, people with EDs report greater sensitivity to other sensory inputs, including touch and sound, which highlights the importance of assessing and treating differences in sensation and perception among those living with EDs (Ingrosso et al., 2024). These data are often linked to a growing body of literature demonstrating overlap between EDs and autism spectrum disorders. Thomas et al. (2024) extend this understanding by emphasizing how neurodivergent individuals, particularly those with autism, experience sensory and interoceptive differences that intersect with body image, food aversions, and emotional regulation. Their narrative review, grounded in lived experience, highlights the importance of recognizing neurodivergence and intersectionality as central to understanding and treating EDs.

People with EDs tend to have different body perception and awareness. With the exception of ARFID as it is currently defined in the DSM-5-TR, fears of gaining weight, perceiving the body as larger than it actually is, and/or pervasive body dissatisfaction are defining diagnostic criteria. Body image itself is considered to be a multisensory experience, driven by specific operations in the brain that include the visual cortex, the insula, and the somatosensory cortex. Current research demonstrates that body disturbances are sensory-processing difficulties, rather than primary thought disturbances. Decades of research have shown that people with EDs have poor interoceptive awareness (IA; Nunn et al., 2008).

IA is a brain-based process that guides how people experience and interpret signals from the body. This brain-body connection is essential for survival because it alerts us to hunger and fullness cues, physical pain, and other sensory and emotional changes in the body. When this process is disrupted, as it is for many with EDs, the act of feeding oneself, moderating pain, and accurately integrating bodily cues is impaired. IA is thought to be processed by the insula, a region of the brain that has been implicated in the development and maintenance of EDs (Nunn et al., 2008). Research on perception from the broader field of neuroscience has shown a link between body image and changes to the parietal lobe and somatosensory cortex. Both brain regions have been shown to influence how people experience the size and shape of their body and how damage to these regions can result in significant differences in body perception.

For instance, a phenomenon known as Alice in Wonderland Syndrome (AIWS) has been observed in people with migraines, epilepsy, and certain brain injuries (Mastria, Mancini, Cesare et al., 2021). AIWS caused by damage to the parietal lobe can cause people to experience their bodies as shrinking or expanding (Friedrich et al., 2024; Mastria et al., 2016). These same brain regions have been implicated in the development and maintenance of EDs (Gadsby, 2017, 2018; Pirton et al., 2018; Uher et al., 2005). Taken together, the biology of sensation and perception in EDs is complex and often not well integrated into traditional treatments that tend to approach body image and sensory difficulties from a purely cognitive lens. We have found that helping clients gain a better understanding of the neurobiology of body image and food preferences is experienced as validating and increases commitment to treatment goals.

## Reward and Threat Sensitivity

Different regions of the brain are responsible for the extent to which a person is motivated by reward and punishment, their degree of impulsivity, and the manner in which the brain detects and processes threat (Zhao et al., 2024). In fact, new data has linked excessive habit formation and the compulsive self-starvation seen in people with anorexia nervosa with low levels of acetylcholine, a neurotransmitter associated with the brain's reward system (Favier et al., 2024). Low reward sensitivity and a compulsive, brain-based drive to restrict food intake means that food, eating, intimacy, socializing, and/or taking risks are significantly less gratifying and the desire to approach is greatly reduced. This may help to explain why some people don't feel a strong inclination toward food or have great difficulty breaking habits, even well into recovery. For those with high reward sensitivity, the brain is reinforced by excitement, novelty, sensation-seeking, and taking chances (Martinelli et al., 2024). This means that food may be experienced as more desirable and harder to avoid. This can also present as boredom later on in treatment when the "usual rewards" (e.g., ED symptoms, higher-risk behaviors) are stabilized but the brain continues to desire heightened stimulation.

Sensitivity to punishment or to aversive stimuli is also related to ED urges and behaviors. Research has identified brain-based systems (e.g., the behavioral inhibition system) that stimulate avoidant behavior in response to punishment. Individuals sensitive to punishment tend to avoid risky options and prioritize avoiding negative consequences over seeking rewards (Eneva, Murray, O'Garro-Moore, J. et al., 2017). For example, when faced with a choice, they may opt for a safer but less rewarding option to minimize potential harm. In the ED context, this may present as extreme rigidity or caution around food intake or weight gain.

## Emotion Regulation Differences

Beyond Linehan's original conceptualization of BPD, unique difficulties with emotion regulation have been well-documented as a transdiagnostic factor in the development of EDs. Individuals with EDs are more likely to have difficulty identifying, communicating, and regulating emotions, and to misread the emotional communication of others. The neuropsychological concept of alexithymia has been studied as a transdiagnostic factor related to ED development and maintenance (Nowakowski et al., 2013; Westwood et al., 2017). Alexithymia is related to functional brain regions including the amygdala, insula, cingulate cortex, parietal lobe, and temporal cortex.

It is essential to situate the ED within the genetic, metabolic, sensory, and other biological influences from which they arise and are maintained. Our clients tell us that this expanded and neurobiologically based understanding is very helpful in making sense of their struggles. When we explain the "bio" part of the theory to our clients, we find that they appreciate visual diagrams such as the one we provide in Figure 3.2.

It can be helpful to provide this figure to your client and ask them to make notes in each quadrant in terms of how their unique life experience fits.

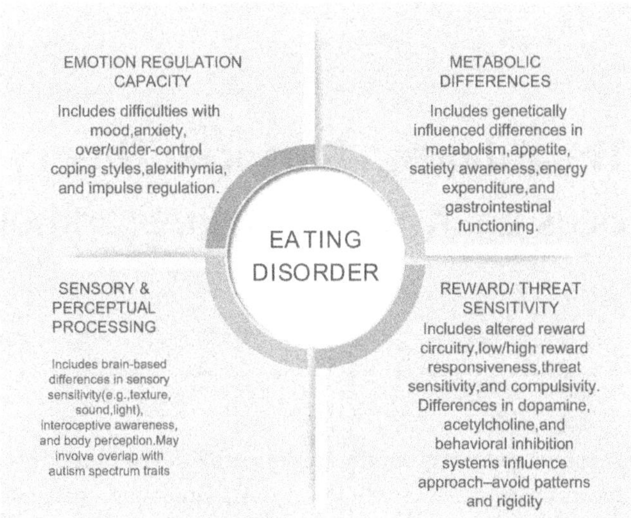


**FIGURE 3.2** The bio-temperamental context of eating disorders. Copyright © 2026 Anita Federici and Lucene Wisniewski. Reprinted by permission.

## Summary

The adapted biosocial theory is used to explain how symptoms arise and are maintained for those with multidiagnostic ED presentations. It is a non-blaming model that emphasizes the transactional nature between biology and environment and is designed to be an engaging and reciprocal discussion with clients. While biological factors help explain the intensity and persistence of ED symptoms, they represent only part of the picture. In the next chapter, we turn our attention to the social and environmental forces—particularly chronic invalidation—that interact with these vulnerabilities to shape the unique clinical profiles we see in MED-DBT.

# 4

# The Adapted Biosocial Theory
## A Focus on Invalidating Environments

Biological vulnerability may set the stage for the development of an eating disorder, but it rarely tells the whole story. As Bulik and colleagues (2005) have described, eating disorders emerge from complex interactions between genetic vulnerability and environmental exposure. To truly understand multidiagnostic ED presentations, we must build upon the neurobiological foundations outlined in Chapter 3 and now zoom out to examine the environmental forces that interact with biology in powerful, often invisible, ways. As Linehan (1993) proposed for borderline personality disorder, chronic invalidation can shape not only how individuals learn to regulate emotions but also how they relate to food, body, identity, and help-seeking over time.

Problems arise due to repeated transactions between biology and an invalidating environment. In addition to the types of invalidation described in the previous chapter, individuals with EDs face unique and pervasive forms of invalidation that are not included in the original DBT framework. For this reason, the biosocial theory needs to be adapted to include environments that chronically invalidate the way a person looks, eats, moves, how much they weigh, and/or how they think, act, and feel about food and their body. Some of these experiences will occur early on in a person's development, while others may occur later on in the course of the ED (e.g., invalidation from healthcare providers).

When teaching this part of the model to clinicians, we have observed discomfort and tension at times, as many recognize things they might have said or done that fall into the categories we describe below. A colleague sent an email after a training to say she felt great shame for having engaged in behaviors in her role as an ED therapist that she now sees were invalidating.

Another physician called to say she felt embarrassed because she didn't know about the sensory or perceptual differences discussed in the adapted biosocial theory and thus had never known how they impacted feeding and body image. She said she felt she had been invalidating many of her patients when assuming that they weren't eating because of a fear of gaining weight. To all of our colleagues who we know are working so hard to deliver support and care to our clients, our response is that we are glad you are willing to be vulnerable and to share these thoughts and feelings with us: it is easy to avoid or suppress them. We have also had many "OMG, I've done that too" moments as we have learned about genetics and neuroscience, invalidation environments, and have listened to those with lived experience. MED-DBT teaches us that we are all doing our best given our own biology and learning histories, *and* we have to do better. Being open to learning and staying connected to current research is how we do better.

Recent work by Downs and colleagues (2025) emphasizes that invalidating environments extend beyond families and interpersonal experiences to broader systems that stigmatize and marginalize individuals with EDs. Historically, knowledge production in the ED field has prioritized certain narratives while excluding others, contributing to epistemic injustice and reinforcing chronic invalidation. Understanding these forces is crucial to fully conceptualizing the environmental contributions to symptom maintenance in MED-DBT. We use the following categories to discuss the MED-DBT additions to the "social" part of the theory (see Figure 4.1).

## Diet Culture

Defined as the glorification of thin, fit (and typically White, cisgender bodies), or thin-thick body ideals, and the rejection of larger bodies, diet culture permeates most aspects of our daily lives. Diet culture refers to both negative attitudes about large bodies and the obsession with thinness/fitness, and to the erroneous belief that health and wellness is a function of body size. Diet culture can be overt (e.g., weight-based teasing) or covert and sometimes out of a person's immediate awareness (as in the case of a person who says they accept all bodies but fears gaining weight themselves or someone who holds implicit biases that people with larger bodies are less motivated or lack willpower).

For those already primed to develop an ED by virtue of their neurobiology, the ubiquitous messaging that self-worth, moral virtue, and/or

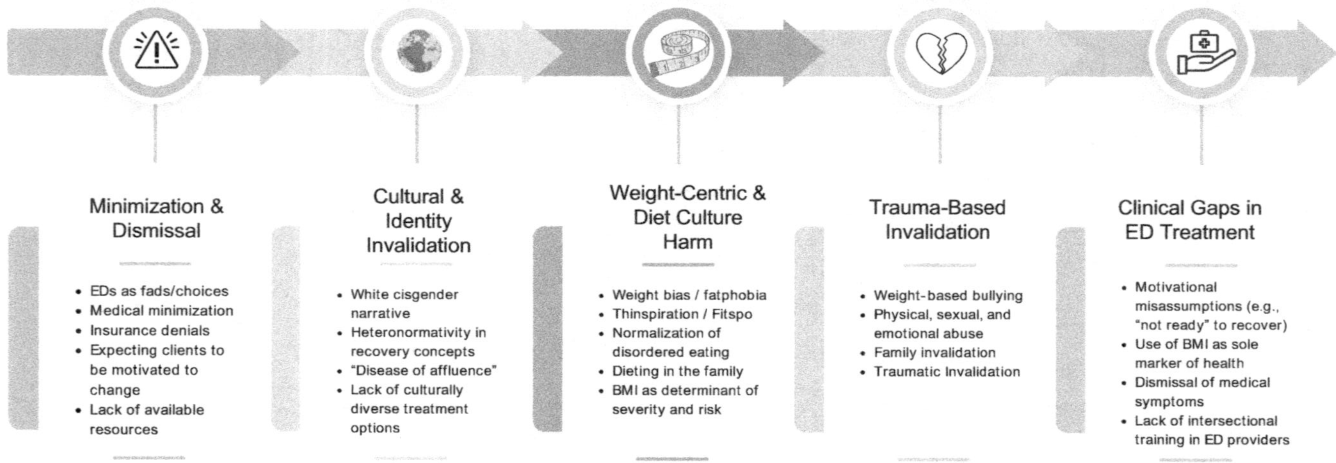


**FIGURE 4.1** Invalidating systems contributing to eating disorders. Copyright © 2026 Anita Federici and Lucene Wisniewski. Reprinted by permission.

success are a function of body shape and weight is incredibly damaging (Alberga et al., 2016). Dieting itself has been shown to be a strong predictor of ED symptoms (Kramer et al., 2024). One young man we worked with painfully described how his older sibling told him he was fat and that nobody loved him throughout his childhood and adolescence. He described being an emotionally sensitive child and the only one in the family living in a larger body. He detailed years of being put on diets by his parents, not allowed to eat birthday cake at parties, and being told that he was lazy and should be more fit like his siblings. He started to diet and exercise at age 14, and within 4 months, he lost so much weight that he was barely recognizable when he returned to school after summer break. His subsequent year in a smaller body was met with significant social reinforcement, inclusion, and dating opportunities. When he was in the pretreatment phase of MED-DBT, he expressed, "If I gain weight by normalizing my eating, all of this (friends, girlfriend, success in sport) will go away and I can't risk that."

The pressure to diet and conform to societal beauty norms begins early in most cultures. Weight and shape-based teasing haunts schoolyards and runs rampant on social media (Cerolini et al., 2024), and fat-phobic attitudes exist in all sectors of business and healthcare (Giel et al., 2010). These are all sources of invalidation. With respect to school settings, invalidation has included the following:

- BMI status listed on report cards
- Weighing kids in gym class
- Teachers labeling food in children's packed lunches as good or bad
- Sending home an option for parents to purchase "slim wear" and "shapewear" to reduce body image distress in youth
- Inaction on the part of teachers/school boards in response to weight-based bullying
- Teaching kids that weight is a function of motivation

Diet culture is also embedded in most medical and healthcare settings (Lawrence et al., 2021). Physicians, on average, receive less than five hours of any training in EDs yet receive many hours of education, workshops, and instruction on treating obesity. Unfortunately, the prevailing view in most medical settings is that lower body weights are healthier and larger bodies are the cause of numerous medical conditions (Ralph et al., 2022). Given that EDs occur across the weight spectrum, diet culture has led to many

EDs being missed, minimized, and, in some cases, reinforced. Examples of invalidation due to diet culture in medical and psychiatric settings include the following:

- Perpetuating the belief that those in larger bodies are unhealthy, lazy, lacking motivation
- Recommendation for weight loss or bariatric surgery without assessing for an ED
- Assuming that most weight loss is positive
- Assuming that only patients with low weights should be taken seriously
- Offering chairs and medical supplies (e.g., gowns, blood pressure cuffs) that only accommodate smaller bodies
- Refusing to treat medical conditions until a patient loses weight

The near-constant advice to diet or treat ailments with medication, intermittent fasting, or surgery is harmful, and to do so in the absence of assessing for the presence of an ED is doubly problematic. The negative psychological and physical effects of weight cycling and weight discrimination are well documented but infrequently discussed with patients. Messages that bodies must be changed and modified to conform to societal standards are often supported by large medical organizations. For instance, the American Pediatric Association recently published updated guidelines calling for aggressive action to be taken for children and teens who are "overweight." This means that families are increasingly being pressured to help their kids lose weight, reinforcing the idea that thinness is healthier, even though this is not supported in the literature. Diet culture upholds the belief that a narrowly defined body type is ideal while discriminating against bodies that do not conform.

Our clients often come from families who also fear weight gain and who themselves engage in dieting behaviors. It is not uncommon for parents to have been bullied or teased about weight and shape themselves and want to avoid a similar experience for their child. One client who would do quite well in treatment when she was away at university would struggle upon her return home because her family was not able to supply the foods she needed on her meal plan. They questioned why she needed to eat breakfast when intermittent fasting was "healthier" and practiced by everyone else in the family. The experience of growing up in a family that places importance on thinness and fitness and communicates negative beliefs about larger bodies is invalidating for the person who struggles to accept themselves as they are and who seeks to recover from the ED.

There is growing recognition of the racialized origins of diet culture (Strings, 2019), the medical misuse of BMI, and the unique ways body image ideals negatively impact BIPOC and LGBTQ2S+ communities (Sonneville & Lipson, 2018). Working against weight stigma and diet culture and advocating for equality and equity for those most marginalized is important in the conceptualization of their illness—and are key treatment targets for building a life worth living.

## Denial of the Problem

Despite increased awareness and education about the genetics and neurobiology of EDs, many families, peers, coaches, schools, insurance companies, and healthcare providers continue to believe EDs are choices or fads. On one end of the continuum, EDs are thought of as deliberate and rebellious acts or means of "attention-seeking." Some people take the position that the ED could be "cured" if the person just "ate already" and "stopped their nonsense." One parent reported that their daughter, who passed away after a 12-year battle with anorexia, was told by a Resident in Emergency that she couldn't come back unless she was ready to get help. Another family described how hard it was to be taken seriously even with a diagnosis, saying their GP told them on diagnosis: "'I know how to treat her. Send her to Africa so she can see what starving children really look like.' Needless to say, we knew we needed a new GP! Our daughter still experiences trauma from that comment."

Such perspectives are also observed across most insurance providers who have repeatedly denied claims for ED treatment on the basis that they are not biological illnesses or valid conditions to qualify for insurance coverage. These types of assumptions are very dangerous and invalidate both the lived experience of those who have an ED and the literature on them. One does not choose an ED any more than one chooses cancer, schizophrenia, or type 1 diabetes. As discussed earlier, ED behaviors soothe an unsettled biology and manage an invalidating environment. The communication that one should "just eat already" is like telling someone with schizophrenia to "just stop hallucinating." Denial or minimization is not only emotionally painful but also confusing for those living with these conditions, who may begin to deny the problem even to themselves.

On the other hand, in families and cultures that celebrate or identify with thinness or fitness, ED behaviors may be viewed as normative and not problematic. For example, a young man who came to treatment due to anorexia struggled because his father, a competitive skier and coach, denied his son's illness, stating he was "just fit and a competitive athlete" like him. Despite his emaciated state and medical instability, his father argued that he was genetically small-boned and thin and biologically able to maintain very low heart rates.

## Medical Minimization

An extension of the previous category, this section refers to invalidation that clients experience when seeking help from medical professionals. This can occur in generalist (non-ED) settings as well as within ED treatment programs. Given (as noted) that most physicians have had almost no ED-specific training, it is not surprising that these illnesses are misunderstood and underdiagnosed in the broader medical community (Kazdin et al., 2017; Seah et al., 2017). In our experience, it is not uncommon for physicians to deny requests for lab work (we have been told on many occasions that it was a waste of resources) or to entirely dismiss or reinforce abnormal vitals (e.g., a patient with a heart rate of 38 beats per minute was told that they had the heart of an athlete). In a recent study of primary physicians' experiences, Tse et al. (2022) highlighted how a lack of training in EDs and weight science leads to biases and assumptions that are harmful to our patients. On reflecting on their own biases, one physician in this publication stated, "I had a patient who came in and told me that she was vomiting and binging and purging, but her weight was fine . . . it took me a while to really believe that she had an eating disorder." Further contributing to this picture, Thompson-Brenner et al. (2012) found that clinicians frequently report feeling frustrated, overwhelmed, and helpless when working with patients with eating disorders, which may contribute to distancing or invalidating responses during treatment.

Over the course of our work, we have collected numerous examples of medical minimization. One individual reported the following:

"ER experiences have always been the worst for me. I had one ER doc tell me I wasn't sick enough to be having heart issues (went in for chest pain that was radiating to my back and down my left arm) . . . any time I bring up my history of an ED when being triaged, most nurses get a look on their face and there's an attitude change. I always avoided going as much as possible."

And a mother wrote to us with the following:

"When we first took our daughter to the family doctor to be assessed/diagnosed, he told us that she wasn't sick enough to require immediate treatment. When I requested bloodwork, because I had been told that most outpatient programs required it, he told me he didn't think we needed it and that it wouldn't likely show anything anyway. I pushed and he agreed to give us a requisition. Two weeks later my daughter got into a new inpatient program. When we went in for the assessment, the doctor in charge told us we couldn't leave because she was too sick. My daughter was hospitalized immediately. Her average resting heart rate was 35 BPM at night for the first three nights in the hospital and a few times it dropped as low as 28 BPM. If I hadn't pushed for the bloodwork and the referral to the new ED program that a friend had told me about, we would still be waiting for help, and my daughter would likely be dead."

In the MED-DBT protocol, it is important to ask about and weave in the way in which these experiences cause, maintain, and/or exacerbate symptoms. Unfortunately, our own ED programs and providers can also maintain invalidating beliefs, behaviors, or systems. For instance, using BMI to define recovery ("I looked better physically but was probably at my sickest") or to determine eligibility for program entry is invalidating (e.g., clients with anorexia or binge-eating disorder turned away from higher levels of care due to "weight being in the average or above average range"). One woman with "atypical" anorexia who had been admitted to a higher level of care reported that she was treated differently in higher levels of care due to her weight: "Even after losing 45% of my weight in a few months, my symptoms were believed to be less severe because I was in the 'normal weight range'. I was told not to gain weight or that concerns about fainting were just anxiety. My family doctor said there was no point in referring back to ED programs because I went and it didn't work." Another client said that when she was hospitalized for ED treatment, a provider said to her, "it's a shame you're here, you just had so much potential."

## Trauma

Having an ED is a traumatic experience in its own right. These are illnesses that threaten one's life and sense of safety. Some patients have been close to death several times. Others have been involuntarily admitted to programs for refeeding. Many have been chemically and physically restrained by hospital staff and sometimes by parents (Downs, 2024b; Downs & Mycock, 2022). Individuals with EDs also experience higher incidences of emotional, physical, and sexual abuse compared to those without EDs, especially those with binge eating and/or purging behaviors. National samples have shown rates of PTSD to be estimated between 20% and 37%, and 50% in those seeking higher levels of care (Dansky et al., 1997; Day et al., 2024). The role of emotional invalidation as well as racial, gender-biased, and oppressive systems have been less recognized in the development of the ED. However, many of our clients' experiences are consistent with Harned's (2022) description of traumatic invalidation.

## Socioeconomic Status and Religious or Cultural Practices

For many people, the ED develops in a context of pervasive psychosocial barriers related to eating, health, and body weight. Those in lower income brackets are more likely to experience food insecurity, have limited access to a variety of foods, and are less likely to access medical services. When they do present for assessment or treatment, they are more likely to experience longer wait times, receive lower levels of care, and not be assessed for an ED compared to those of higher socioeconomic status (Kazdin et al., 2017). The long-standing myth that EDs are "diseases of affluence" contributes to biases by healthcare providers (Huryk et al., 2021) and represents an important source of invalidation for our clients. Socioeconomic status is also linked to racial and ethnic disparities that uniquely impact ED development and maintenance (Burke et al., 2020). Unequal resources, inadequate access to evidence-based assessment and treatment, being treated as different from others, marginalization, and oppression are invalidating environments that our clients experience that are typically not discussed in dominant ED frameworks.

It is also important to consider the influence of religion, cultural identity, and spirituality. While these play important roles in recovery and life worth living goals, at times, the expectation to rigidly adhere to customs, rituals, and ceremonies can be experienced as invalidating. Most religions observe periods of fasting or food restriction (e.g., Lent, Ramadan), others have specific views about appearance and the way one "should" look (e.g., modest dress/clothing for Muslim women, pressure to look/act a certain way for marriage ceremonies in Orthodox Jewish communities). Of particular note are cultural and spiritual practices that emphasize going without, self-punishment, sexual repression, and heteronormativity. While these practices do not cause EDs on their own, they can form part of an environment that disallows diversity or nonconformity.

The impact of chronic invalidation is substantive: in theory, it exacerbates the underlying biotemperament and facilitates the development and maintenance of the ED. As stated, these conversations can be uncomfortable for clients, families, and clinicians. But as difficult as these topics may be, we have found that they significantly increase engagement in treatment. As providers, when we acknowledge how our treatments have been invalidating, commitment increases. Communicating that the client makes sense is validating. Validation calms the threat system and creates space for you and your client to accurately hear one another.

## Putting It All Together

Explaining these theoretical details can be overwhelming for both client and therapist. Keep in mind that the biosocial theory will be discussed repeatedly over the course of treatment to aid in familiarity and application. In our experience, clients feel energized by the adapted biosocial theory. The goal of explaining it is to help the client make sense of their struggles and to demonstrate how the collision between biology and environment created the "perfect storm" for the ED to develop. It is critical for the client to recognize themselves in the model in order to pursue MED-DBT. In this way, the adapted biosocial theory serves as a blueprint to aid in self-discovery and provides the roadmap for a new path forward.

## Case Study: Sara

Sara is a 27-year-old cisgender female. She has been diagnosed with AN-B/P, PTSD, ADHD, alcohol and cocaine abuse, and BPD. She was recently discharged from a residential ED program due to lack of behavioral change with respect to the ED and due to ongoing suicidal and self-injurious behavior. She was able to stop using substances while in the program.

## Presenting Issues

- Chronic suicidal and self-injurious thinking and planning (present most days), three previous suicide attempts, cutting at least once per week, multiple scarring on wrists, arms, thighs, and stomach. Reports that self-injury is a harm reduction strategy to cope with emotions and to stop herself from engaging in suicidal behavior. Says she cannot address weight gain or eating more without self-injury being available.
- ED symptoms: Current BMI = 17.4. Subjective binge episodes two times per week. Self-induced vomiting two to five times per week. Excessive exercise five days per week, including walking, running, skipping, and weight training. Current labs show medical stability, though a review of labs over the previous six weeks shows bradycardia, orthostatic hypotension, and hypokalemia.
- Mood is described as labile "but better when my weight is lower."
- She has stopped using drugs and alcohol though noted that she is having significant urges to use again.
- Client reports occasional shoplifting and risky sexual behaviors that lead to shame and overall increase in symptoms.

### Background

- Sara was "anxious" and sensitive as a child, restless, bored easily, had a hard time paying attention in school. She described herself as "emotionally all over the place" from a young age, often experiencing intense emotions and fears of abandonment.
- She noted that her father has anger issues, mother is a people pleaser. She was always trying to keep the peace, feared conflict.
- A half-brother was diagnosed with schizophrenia. She described her older and younger sisters as high achievers, good at school, and accomplished in their careers. She said that her father, when upset with her, would ask her why she couldn't be more like her sisters. She thinks her younger sister has an eating disorder.
- Sensory issues were noted at an early age with respect to textures of food, sounds, and touch. High disgust reflex. Body image distress started prior to sexual assault as she recalls always feeling like her body didn't match her sense of herself, like she was "wearing someone else's body."

- Pervasive diet talk in the family, fat phobia, and glorification of thin/fit body ideals.
- Parents had difficulty with the way Sara ate and with her emotional lability. They described her as "attention-seeking" and dramatic and "not at all like her sisters." Mom wondered what she "did wrong" with Sara to make her so different.
- At age 12, she started experimenting with marijuana and alcohol and felt more social and less anxious when using.
- At age 13, she started dieting and had a strong desire to lose weight.
- At age 14, she was sexually assaulted at a party. Although she went to the police, she was interviewed by three male officers who challenged her memory and she left feeling confused and not believed. Her peers at school blamed her for the assault and told her she should stop talking about it. This led to her first suicide attempt.
- The years following the sexual assault were tumultuous. She said that "everything just intensified." She restricted her food intake to one small meal per day and started running. She lost a significant amount of weight by age 15 and was hospitalized due to medical instability. Her parents and grandparents often argued over how "difficult" she was being with respect to ED treatment and often grew angry during meal support for her unwillingness to eat "like normal people."
- Between the ages of 15 and 19, Sara was hospitalized in ED day treatment four times and admitted to general psychiatry units six times for suicidal ideation. During these years, she began to binge eat and purge, sometimes three times per day for many months, resulting in greater medical instability.
- Her parents grew frustrated with the lack of treatment progress and felt that she wasn't trying hard enough to get better.
- Notes from psychiatric treatment programs described Sara as "borderline," "manipulative," and "not motivated to change."

## Biosocial Theory Step-by-Step

- **Step 1:** Describe the "bio" part of the biosocial theory, emphasizing both the genetics and neurobiology of eating disorders as well as information on emotion regulation processes.

- **Step 2:** Demonstrate which parts of Sara's personal history are in line with the biological aspects of the model. For example, she described being an anxious and sensitive child with intense emotions. She was bored easily and has a history of engaging in risk-taking behaviors. These factors may point to an underlying emotional sensitivity and differences in reward sensitivity and inhibitory mechanisms. There is also a family history of schizophrenia (recent articles highlight a potential shared genetic etiology between schizophrenia and anorexia), anger management issues with her father, and a possible ED with respect to her sister. These are important factors in understanding the biology of Sara's ED. Her strong disgust mechanism, sensory issues, and body disturbances have been associated with differences in accompanying brain regions. When teaching clients about their biotemperaments, it is important to emphasize that there is no such thing as a "good" versus "bad" temperament. Rather, everyone's brain is organized in a unique way. Part of recovery is understanding how our brain works, so more effective life and treatment decisions can be made.

  Sometimes clients will initially report feeling hopeless when hearing about their biology and genetics, thinking that this is something they cannot change. However, in our experience, knowing how to work with your biology (as opposed to against it or not even knowing how it works) is much more likely to lead to a better outcome. During discussions about brain and genetics, we highlight positive and adaptive aspects of one's biology. For Sara, it is important for her to know that the world needs people who are risk-takers, creative thinkers, sensation-seekers, and who are willing to do things differently. What it also means is that Sara's symptoms have likely reinforced those characteristics. For example, purging, starvation, shoplifting, and self-injury can be especially rewarding and likely satisfy her biological need to be busy and stimulated. This is possibly one reason she feels so bored and restless in the recovery phases of treatment. She doesn't know how to work with her biology differently and ultimately returns to what worked in the past. During the pretreatment phase with Sara, we agreed that one of her treatment targets would need to be finding ways to cope with boredom since this was a big factor related to relapse and symptom initiation.

- **Step 3:** Explain the "social" of the biosocial theory with respect to invalidation of emotional experience as well as invalidation as it relates to body, weight, food, and eating. Sara described a number of invalidating experiences across her developmental history including sexual assault, being disbelieved and dismissed by police and peers, frequent comparisons to her sisters, diet culture within the family home, feeling blamed by parents and providers that she wasn't succeeding in treatment, being told to be like "normal" people around food, misunderstanding the sensory and perceptual differences she experienced, communicating that she was making choices in terms of her actions, assuming that she could do it differently if she tried harder, and being told that wanting attention is abnormal. It is necessary to help Sara see that she is not just coping with her biology but with environments that have been pervasively invalidating.

- **Step 4:** Check that the model fits with Sara's lived experience. The idea is to help your client see that "all behavior is caused"—that it has been developed, practiced, and reinforced for many years. You will work to normalize and validate that Sara's ways of coping make sense. She is not crazy, bad, manipulative, or too difficult. Your job is to communicate "how could it be otherwise," given her biology and learning history.
- **Step 5:** Use an example from the client's recent past in which they engaged in a behavior. Using the model of emotion dysregulation (Figure 4.2), work together to highlight vulnerability factors, the

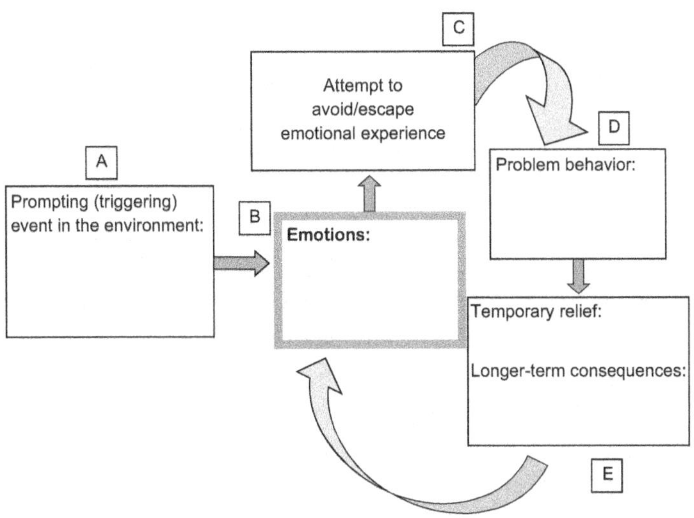


**FIGURE 4.2** The model of emotion dysregulation. From Safer (2018). Copyright © 2018 The Guilford Press. Reprinted by permission.

prompting event, emotions, and how the symptom helped the client cope with their biology and/or the invalidating environment. Discuss that this overlearned pattern, rooted in biology and learning history, leads to temporary relief. Also discuss that the problem is not the client, but that the client hasn't been given opportunities to learn how to work with their unique neurobiology and navigate pervasive invalidation; this leaves them perpetually more vulnerable the next time they must face adversity. The outcome of this pattern is that the client exists on an "emotional hamster wheel," running to avoid but not actually moving anywhere.

When working through this with Sara, she discussed a recent episode when she was in the hospital in which she was physically restrained after becoming very dysregulated in the kitchen. She reported the following:

- Vulnerability factors: poor sleep (4–5 hours), malnourished, did not take medication as prescribed
- Trigger: Walking into the kitchen and seeing that there was pasta for lunch (feared food)
- Emotions: Fear, disgust (primary), anger (secondary)
- Attempt to reduce/avoid painful emotions: started screaming, ran out of the kitchen, yelled, "I will not eat that. I would rather be dead." Ran into the group room and started to bang her head against the wall. This led to physical and chemical restraint on the unit.
- Temporary relief: didn't have to eat the pasta, felt "in control" by not eating, felt "powerful" because the team couldn't force her to eat, pain of hitting her head felt "satisfying" and distracted her from fear and disgust.

- **Step 6:** Check in and consolidate. Is this making sense to your client? What are we missing? Does the biosocial theory fit with their lived experience? Ask your client to continue to reflect on their experiences for homework so you can continue to expand and develop the model together.

## Summary

In our experience, clients report feeling understood, empowered, hopeful, and more willing to engage in the MED-DBT program given the way symptoms are presented and explained. Thus, this type of collaborative case conceptualization is the backbone of the treatment model and a powerful first step in building commitment to the overall treatment plan

Together, the biological and environmental factors outlined in Chapters 3 and 4 offer a comprehensive and compassionate understanding of how multidiagnostic EDs develop and persist. The adapted biosocial theory recognizes that ED symptoms do not develop at random l, but rather emerge from the intersection of biological sensitivities, sustained patterns of invalidation and attempts to manage thoughts and emotions. For clients who have felt misunderstood, mistreated, or mislabeled by previous care systems, this framework can begin to restore hope and clarity. As we transition into Chapter 5, we turn our attention to the foundational treatment assumptions that shape how we deliver MED-DBT. These assumptions are not just abstract ideals—they are practical tools that help us counteract the very invalidation our clients have internalized, and they guide us in staying grounded, principled, and effective throughout the therapeutic process.

# 5

# Assumptions about MED-DBT Clients

In MED-DBT, how we conceptualize our clients is not an afterthought—it is foundational. Assumptions shape how we understand behaviors, interpret engagement, and ultimately determine the direction of treatment. This chapter outlines the core treatment assumptions adapted from standard DBT and applied specifically to clients with multidiagnostic eating disorders. These assumptions are more than philosophical ideals; they are actionable principles that help us stay grounded, nonjudgmental, and effective in the face of complexity. To illustrate their practical significance, we begin with a clinical example that highlights how different assumptions can shape entirely different treatment paths.

## Case Study: Sasha

Sasha is a 24-year-old client diagnosed with anorexia nervosa—binge/purge type (AN-B/P) and BPD. In the last 16 months, she has been admitted to ED day treatment programs three times with little success and had four ER visits for suicidality and/or being unable to eat, leading to medical instability. In reviewing her treatment records, it is noted that day treatment admissions were marked by increased self-injury, suicidal communication, "refusal" to enter the kitchen, screaming at staff when asked to eat, and crying loudly and strongly uncontrollably. Sasha had been seen by several outpatient therapists trialing FBT, CBT-ED, and supportive models. A review of her file shows that her notes detailing a lack of agreement on treatment goals, nonattendance, incomplete homework, and withdrawal or anger when pushed to change. Thus, the outpatient history shows early termination or the therapist "firing her" or telling her she needs a higher level of care.

How you think about your client matters. Your interpretation and the assumptions you make regarding Sasha's behavior will influence her treatment journey. Let's take a look at two possible conceptualizations of this case. We will then discuss how this relates to the DBT treatment assumptions.

## Conceptualization 1

You believe that Sasha is looking for attention. You conceptualize her behaviors as a reflection of "poor parenting" and formulate Sasha's difficulties as cognitive in nature. You assume that Sasha has control over how she manages her emotions and behaviors but is choosing to "act out" instead. You view past therapy attempts as evidence that Sasha does not want to get better, and you are leaning toward not offering her treatment at this time.

## Conceptualization 2

You explain to your team (and to the client) that Sasha's behaviors make sense given the pervasive neurometabolic mechanisms that drive anorexia as well as the biology that underlies the emotion regulation and interpersonal deficits that characterize BPD. For example, you believe that Sasha would be highly triggered by attempts to eat *and* not know how to regulate herself. In this way, you also recognize how Sasha has been shaped by culture and environment. You wonder if self-injury has been reinforced as a short-term way to distract from intense emotions. As well, Sasha has a long history of people backing off when she screams and sobs or when she shuts down, leading you to be curious about how her behavior has played an important functional role for her and in the management of the ED.

Your conceptualization drives treatment decisions and all of your interactions with your client. How might the treatment progress for the clinician who proposes conceptualization 1? What about for the clinician who puts forward conceptualization 2?

If a clinician holds the first conceptualization of Sasha—as manipulative, resistant, and responsible for her own suffering—they are likely to withhold treatment or offer it with limited warmth, engagement, or flexibility. This often leads to rupture, early dropout, or reinforcement of the client's internalized invalidation and hopelessness. In contrast, a clinician grounded in the second conceptualization will see Sasha's behaviors as making sense in the context of neurobiological vulnerability and learned survival strategies. Treatment would begin by validating the presence of these behaviors while still targeting their function and reinforcing alternative, skillful responses. This stance allows the therapist to stay curious, collaborative, and nonjudgmental—essential ingredients in building trust and promoting change.

MED-DBT, like standard DBT, is a principle-driven (as opposed to protocol-driven) treatment that maximizes flexibility (Linehan, 1993). Treatment decisions are based on your knowledge and fluid use of the theories and assumptions that underlie this model. In this chapter, we describe how Linehan's (1993) treatment assumptions about clients are applied in MED-DBT. These assumptions counter the invalidating environments our clients are accustomed to, help providers stay out of emotion mind, and reduce judgmental or pejorative formulations of a client's behavior. When unsure of how to proceed in treatment, MED-DBT treatment assumptions provide direction. If we can help you approach these complicated, multidiagnostic cases while offering MED-DBT at the highest level possible and in a way that maintains your energy and commitment to the process, we feel that we have succeeded in something important. The DBT assumptions are an important part of this.

## The MED-DBT Assumptions

### Clients with Multidiagnostic EDs Are Doing the Best They Can

It is not uncommon for providers to believe that clients are not trying hard enough in terms of treatment or recovery. Ambivalence, not following medical recommendations, skipping meals, exercising when bradycardic, or missing appointments are often highlighted as "evidence" that clients are not really doing their best. Some practitioners might believe that if the client really wanted to get better, they would make more of an effort. In MED-DBT, we believe that every client is doing their best given their biotemperament and unique learning histories. The stance, when observing behavior, is one of "*how could it be otherwise*" given the metabolic, sensory, and perceptual disturbances, emotional sensitivity and overactive limbic system, neurodiversity and differences in learning styles, the history of pervasive and traumatic invalidation, and the way in which the environment has responded to these behaviors in the past (see Chapter 4 on the adapted biosocial theory).

At any moment, no matter how egregious a behavior, we believe that clients are doing their best to regulate, stay safe, and avoid threats. With an unsettled biology and a pervasive lack of skills to navigate the world, the behaviors and choices of our clients make a lot of sense. The drive to stay safe and avoid threats is not pathological; we all engage in behavior that maximizes our sense of safety. When we view the actions of our clients in this light (i.e., that everything arises out of a fundamental need for survival and/or regulation), judgments fall away and clinicians are better able to formulate responses and interventions that are compassionate, even when pushing for change.

## Clients Want to Improve

We have treated hundreds of clients and spent years consulting with programs and practitioners around the globe about their patients. To date, we have never met a client who did not want to improve. This is especially striking given that we are often consulted about individuals described as "not wanting to get better," "choosing to stay sick," or some variation of being unmotivated or resistant. Your beliefs and assumptions about whether your client wants to get better significantly influence your approach. If you believe your client is unwilling or uninterested in change, you may unintentionally offer less effort, fewer interventions, and reduced optimism compared to the support you'd give to someone you perceive as motivated.

It is often the case that our clients *do* want to improve, *and* they feel ambivalent about whether changing their ED behaviors is necessary, or even possible, for them to feel better. That is why it is critical to differentiate between a desire to improve and an ability or willingness to change specific behaviors. These concepts are frequently conflated. When we talk about wanting to improve, we refer to the assumption we hold that our clients want to feel better, be at peace, feel more grounded, have a sense of safety, and experience less suffering. We *do not* assume our clients know how to articulate this, believe it is possible for them, or have the skills yet to pursue it.

Our adapted biosocial theory helps explain why it might appear that clients don't want to improve. Often, ED behaviors serve important short-term regulatory functions and may be reinforced by both internal (e.g., emotional relief, numbing, identity stability) and external factors (e.g., increased care or attention when medically unwell, validation from providers following weight loss). Clinicians are therefore urged to separate the desire to improve from the ways a behavior is reinforced. Holding this distinction allows us to remain compassionate and validating while maintaining clinical precision. Together, these first two assumptions challenge the damaging narrative that clients are manipulative, resistant, or uninterested in recovery. Embracing both helps us stay anchored in a nonjudgmental stance, one that honors our clients' struggles while continuing to invite change.

## Clients Need to Do Better, Try Harder, and Be More Motivated to Change

At first, this treatment assumption seems to counter the first two, and sometimes, when teaching this assumption, ED clinicians will say that this feels too harsh or overly judgmental. Keep in mind that no assumption is meant to be applied in isolation of the others. Together with the first two, this assumption represents a core dialectic: we assume that our clients are doing the best they can *and* currently the best they can is not enough to get them the change that they want. We point out to clients that their current ways of coping—restricting, binge eating, purging, nonsuicidal self-injury (NSSI)—and approaching situations (e.g., active passivity, apparent compliance) are likely experienced as helping in the short term but are not compatible with building a life worth living in the long term. If the current efforts were sufficient, the client wouldn't need this treatment! Therefore, although they are working as hard as they can given their situation and the skills that they have currently, they need to do better, try harder, and be more motivated even though what they're doing right now is the best they can do. This is where we come in. Our job is to help them learn new skills and to use them in new contexts and to help them maintain and develop motivation to sustain that change over time.

## Clients Did Not Cause All of Their Problems and They Have to Be Involved in Solving Them Anyway

As outlined in the MED-DBT biosocial theory, EDs and emotion regulation deficits are thought to be caused by biology and pervasive invalidation; they are not choices. Clients do not choose the way their brains operate, how their DNA has been sequenced, or the systems and cultures they were born into. They did not cause the traumas that have befallen them nor are they responsible for environments and systems that failed them, *and* they need to be part of the solution (note again the dialectical thinking!). No problem is solved without some sort of action. If a problem is impacting us, regardless of the origin of the cause, it is ours to solve. This can be very difficult when clients feel strongly that their circumstances are unfair. In the case example at the beginning of the chapter, Sasha did not like this treatment assumption when she learned about it. Given many treatment attempts that she described as unhelpful and often harmful, the notion that she had to be part of solving her problems was upsetting to her ("Why should I have to fix a broken system? You are the expert who should be able to help me."). This last tenet is important because it reminds us that we can help with the solution but we cannot actually solve our clients' problems without them. Here we ask both the client and the clinician to embrace radical responsibility—recognizing that blame has no role in treatment, but accountability is essential for recovery.

## Clients Must Learn New Behaviors in All Relevant Contexts

Generalizing skills outside of the therapy context, or from one level of care to another, is essential. While your client may be able to eat in session with you, use interpersonal skills with the dietitian, or manage medical stability in a residential program, it is imperative that they learn to do these tasks at home, at work/school, and in other social contexts. In their book on DBT, Galen and Aguirre (2021) use a swimming analogy to highlight the spirit of this assumption: Learning to dog paddle may be enough when taking a short swim in the local pool near the shallow end, but it wouldn't be enough for someone caught in a deep lake in the middle of a storm when the wind and the waves are overwhelming. If the client's current skills were sufficient to build a life worth living, they wouldn't need treatment. This is not to suggest that clients don't have any skills; in fact, they have many! It is the fact that different skills are needed or current skills need to be generalized so they can be accessed when urges are high (e.g., eating while with friends on campus, tolerating feeling full outside of session, managing body image distress during a family dinner).

## Clients Cannot Fail MED-DBT Treatment

Our clients come with multiple unsuccessful treatment attempts, and many feel that they have simply failed and/or that they are beyond help. Consistent with standard DBT, the MED-DBT model maintains that clients cannot fail the treatment. When treatment isn't working, it is because we do not have a treatment strategy or alternative methods that might be more effective for a particular person. The treatment can fail but the client cannot. Linehan has said that it is the job of the therapist to know how to treat a patient. It is not the patient's job to know how to treat the problems that brought them to treatment. Yet in mental health, there is a long history of blaming patients for being unwilling, labeling them as treatment resistant, or as unmotivated to change. In contrast, when treatments do not work in medicine it is less common for the patient to be blamed. For example, we don't say that a patient failed chemotherapy or that they were unwilling/ unmotivated when surgery to fix a brain aneurysm is unsuccessful.

When providers take the position that a lack of treatment progress is a failure on the part of the patient, it perpetuates the invalidating environment and demotivates the need to change programs and systems. It communicates that if the patient really wanted to get better, they would, which contradicts the entirety of the biosocial theory. Imagine if cancer researchers concluded that unsuccessful interventions were due to patient motivation and resistance. They would never seek out new treatments because they would believe that they already had all the treatments they needed to cure cancer if, after all, it was simply "treatment-resistant patients" that were to blame. Instead, this assumption helps providers maintain a nonjudgmental framework and drives novel research developments. It was in this context that DBT was developed. Recognizing that patients with BPD were not to blame for their response to treatments, Linehan pioneered the development of a treatment that would change the face of psychiatric care. This wouldn't have been possible if she held the belief that patients fail treatment.

## MED-DBT Clinicians Can Fail in Delivering the Treatment

This assumption tends to garner a fair bit of confusion and emotion from practitioners. How is it that clients can't fail but therapists can? Isn't the word "fail" judgmental? This assumption reminds us that we are fallible and that therapist drift is a common phenomenon. The word "fail" is not intended to be critical, rather to reflect its dictionary meaning: to be unsuccessful in achieving a goal, to neglect to do something, or to observe that something has broken down. Observing this assumption means that we take responsibility for the ways we are not adherent to the model, observe and correct therapy drift, acknowledge the ways we interfere with treatment, and recognize that we can deliver MED-DBT in a way that it was not intended. The high stakes and unique needs of our clients can easily cause even the most skilled and seasoned therapist to stray from the treatment protocol (e.g., targeting body image instead of bradycardia, not addressing water loading as a therapy-interfering behavior, avoiding talking about food monitoring). This assumption invites us to engage in a nonjudgmental and reflective process with our consult teams and to be open to feedback from clients and colleagues about the ways in which we may fail in delivering the treatment.

### Clinicians Working in MED-DBT Need Support

MED-DBT treatment is comprehensive and complex. The people we serve have complicated problems. The clinician is managing a severe neurobiological illness alongside suicidality, emotion dysregulation, trauma, and self-injury. Emotions run high. Pressure from multiple sources can be intense. In addition, guiding clients through treatment requires clinicians to have a solid grasp on their own beliefs and biases about body weight and nutrition. For all of these reasons, this treatment is not designed to be delivered by a solo practitioner. The model requires ongoing consultation to reduce therapist burnout and to increase adherence to the model. Participation in weekly MED-DBT team consultation (as outlined in Chapter 16) is a requirement for those working with this model.

## Summary

The MED-DBT client assumptions are essential tools for staying out of judgment and in wise mind. When fully understood and consistently applied, they act as both a compass and an anchor for the treatment process—keeping clinicians grounded, hopeful, and effective, even when facing highly complex and emotionally charged presentations. These assumptions also serve as a direct response to the invalidation our clients have so often experienced in treatment systems. In the next chapter, we explore the parallel assumptions about clinicians that form the other half of this treatment relationship, and the practices that sustain provider well-being, accountability, and adherence in this high-intensity work.

# 6

# Building Your MED-DBT Team

MED-DBT is a team-based, multidisciplinary, and multimodal treatment; it is not intended to be used by solo practitioners. All team members are trained in the model and accept the theories (e.g., biosocial theory), assumptions about clients (outlined in Chapter 3), and team agreements (described in this chapter) that underlie this approach. MED-DBT theories and assumptions "form the groundwork context on which DBT was built and provide a basis for therapeutic decision-making throughout the treatment" (Linehan, 1993, p. 119). Treatment is most effective when the team voluntarily agrees to work together within the MED-DBT framework. That said, joining a DBT team can be a steep learning curve and a marked shift in approach for those trained in traditional ED approaches and/or working in the context of a medical model. Therefore, it is important to evaluate each team member's interest and willingness to work within the MED-DBT framework before bringing new team members on board.

As depicted in Figure 6.1, you and your client are the central hub of the treatment, working in collaboration with your skills group leaders. In addition, your client will receive treatment from registered dietitians, primary care physicians, and psychiatrists on an as-needed basis. In some cases, these healthcare practitioners will be part of your team. In other cases (see the next section) you and your client will need to coordinate care with outside providers. The team coordinates care such that your client receives the following modalities over a minimum period of 6 months:

- Weekly individual MED-DBT therapy (including phone coaching)
- Weekly skills group training (with different facilitators than the individual therapist)

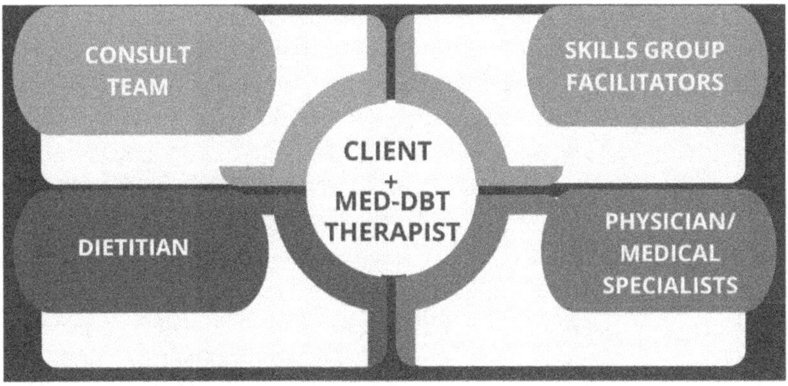


**FIGURE 6.1** The MED-DBT team. Copyright © 2026 Anita Federici and Lucene Wisniewski. Reprinted by permission.

- As-needed meetings with a registered dietitian
- As-needed appointments with a primary health provider and/or psychiatrist
- A therapist who attends weekly consultation team meetings

We recognize that many of you are working on your own, without a team. While it is not feasible for one provider to deliver all aspects of this treatment, it is possible to build partnerships or to recruit providers in your community who can work together to help your client. We appreciate that this might not be an easy task. For example, depending on where you live, it might be very difficult to access primary care and psychiatry. It may also be challenging to recruit physicians into private practice models due to competing demands on their time. In Canada, it has taken us years to recruit a family physician and a psychiatrist to join us, both on a very part-time basis. In the absence of primary care physicians "in house," we have been able to develop strong working relationships with medical providers in our communities. For us, it has meant developing materials and offering phone calls and lunch-and-learn opportunities to explain how our program works and the ways we might work together. Notably, with the expanded use of virtual platforms, we now have access to people who are farther away, which has improved accessibility. We have found that many medical practitioners welcome the collaboration, as the clients have chronic and varied needs that they cannot manage on their own. Similarly, it may be challenging to locate registered dietitians (RDs) to collaborate with, particularly those with ED training and expertise. It is also much more difficult to find RDs with DBT experience, although we are seeing a larger number attending our trainings.

Working with external providers presents unique challenges. The most significant being that they may not be MED-DBT trained and are unlikely to attend your weekly consultation team meetings. This will likely present conflicts about decision making as there will be different philosophies and assumptions operating simultaneously. For instance, you may have a dietitian who focuses on increasing full meal compliance when you are trying to focus on reducing suicidal thinking and self-harm behavior and view meal plan compliance as a quality-of-life-interfering behavior. Likewise, you may have a physician telling your client that they are medically stable with "nothing to worry about" despite a low heart rate at the same time as you are targeting bradycardia as a T1 life-threatening behavior. It is not uncommon for there to be competing views and ideologies about weight goals, weight science, and meal plan goals (see Chapter 9 on targeting in MED-DBT). Different approaches can be therapy-interfering and, therefore, would become a target of the treatment. We recommend orienting external providers as much as possible to the model to maximize collaboration. In these circumstances, it is often a function of the therapy to assist our clients in building a skill set to increase effectiveness around negotiating with ancillary providers (see Chapter 10 on individual sessions in MED-DBT for further discussion).

## Team Agreements: How We Operate in MED-DBT

Just as we do in standard DBT, our protocol requires you and your team to commit to observing the DBT assumptions about clients (see Chapter 3) and practice in a manner that is guided by a set of team agreements. In this section, we present the six original team agreements developed by Linehan (1993), expanded upon by Sayrs (2019), and recently adapted to be more inclusive, diverse, and equitable. For those trained predominantly in traditional ED treatments, these agreements will represent a shift in philosophy and approach. For those trained in standard DBT, we want to demonstrate how these agreements apply to the treatment of complex and multidiagnostic ED presentations.

### Dialectical Agreement

In MED-DBT, we commit to viewing conflicts, contradictions, and differing perspectives as opportunities for synthesis rather than signs of failure.

A dialectical stance means accepting that more than one truth can exist at the same time, and our job is to move forward by integrating those truths. This mindset is especially important in ED work, where historically rigid beliefs about recovery, nutrition, and treatment compliance can clash with the lived experiences of our clients.

As Sayrs (2019) notes, dialectics guides us to search for synthesis when strongly held opposing views threaten to divide the team. Granato et al. (2022) emphasize that adopting a dialectical lens includes acknowledging our biases and working to understand differing viewpoints, particularly those shaped by marginalization. In practice, this means moving away from polarized thinking—for example, EDs are about food versus EDs are not about food—and instead, embracing the tension and using it to guide collaborative decision making. This stance helps prevent provider burnout and protects the therapeutic alliance.

Participating in a MED-DBT team means committing to using dialectics to understand the situations and behaviors of our clients, their families, and our colleagues. We agree that more than one thing can be true at the same time, to move away from "right versus wrong" thinking, and to move forward by seeking a synthesis between opposing views. We lean into confusion, practice throwing ourselves into change, and work to let go of extreme or binary ways of operating. This is especially important when working with EDs, where, historically, there have been narrow views of recovery criteria regarding what constitutes a positive treatment response and little flexibility in terms of pathways to get better. Let's take a look at some common dialectical tensions that are observed in MED-DBT:

- EDs are about food and body weight.
- *EDs are not about food and body weight.*
- Weight and nutritional stability are key treatment goals.
- *Focusing on weight and nutritional stability can be problematic.*
- Gaining weight is an important target when treating EDs.
- *Gaining weight is difficult in a weight-obsessed and fat-phobic culture.*
- EDs affect all genders, cultures, and ages.
- *Most ED programs are geared for White, middle-class, heterosexual, and neurotypical cisgender women.*
- Your client wants to work with you.
- *Your client does not want to address their eating disorder.*

- Psychiatry recommends a higher level of care.
- *You recommend continuing with outpatient MED-DBT.*
- Eating a wide variety of foods is part of ED recovery.
- *Your client has significant sensory and textural difficulties and cannot eat some types/varieties of food.*
- The dietitian recommends following a traditional ED meal plan.
- *The meal plan is not culturally applicable to clients from diverse backgrounds.*

In the absence of a dialectical worldview, you may find yourself becoming polarized with your teammates and your clients about the dialectical tensions that will arise in this treatment. Without a framework for navigating these conflicts, it is easy to feel defensive, emotionally distressed, ineffective, and experience higher burnout. Likewise, our clients also feel disheartened, misunderstood, dysregulated, and less motivated when their perspectives are minimized or viewed as contradictory (and therefore problematic) to the treatment plan. Our patients have reported to us that they commonly feel that their needs for more diverse care pathways, harm reduction models, and better integration of neurodiversity within ED treatment have been "dead-end" conversations often minimized as "This is just your ED talking" by others. It makes sense that managing divergent points of view would be challenging, especially when the work involves clients who may be medically unstable, ambivalent, suicidal, malnourished, and presenting with multiple problem behaviors. These conversations are also magnified by system constraints that include lack of funding, understaffed clinics, teams that are not trained to manage multidiagnostic presentations, and the pressure to admit people quickly into programs. As such, you and your client may find yourselves uncertain of how to move forward.

In MED-DBT, we agree ahead of time to acknowledge that there are multiple truths operating in any given moment. We accept that we operate from our own experiences (which entail specific cultural and gender-based ideologies) and therefore, do not hold the full truth. We agree to move away from right versus wrong thinking styles and instead search for synthesis. For example, instead of becoming polarized with a client who wants to work with you but does not want to increase food and fluid intake, the therapist searches for a middle ground. Can the client agree to stay alive in order to work together as a start (i.e., maintaining medical stability, not losing more weight, taking potassium pills if purging occurs)? While this approach might feel uncomfortable for those trained in traditional ED models, it has been our experience that it is precisely this stance that helps to engage our clients. Please see Chapter 10 for a larger discussion on secondary targets and dialectical dilemmas.

## Consultation-to-the-Client Agreement

This agreement encourages us to help clients build the skills to advocate for themselves, rather than stepping in as intermediaries. The goal is to promote client empowerment by teaching them to address issues directly with other providers when possible, fostering independence and generalization of interpersonal skills. Sayrs (2019) explains that when we intervene for the client, we may deprive them of the opportunity to learn essential problem-solving strategies. Granato et al. (2022) extend this, acknowledging that advocacy may still be necessary in oppressive systems but should be done in tandem with skill-building and without fragilizing the client. We illustrate this with the example of a client upset after a difficult session with their dietitian. Rather than emailing the dietitian on the client's behalf, the therapist collaborated with the client to validate emotions, identify values, and rehearse a DEAR MAN script to resolve the conflict themselves. The result was a moment of growth and restored connection.

During treatment, a client approached her individual session very anxious and angry following a meeting with the team dietitian. The client reported that the dietitian didn't take her concerns seriously, didn't understand that she could not eat the new foods presented on her meal plan, and that she observed the dietitian rolling her eyes during their meeting. The client stated that she did not want to work with the dietitian, was unsure if she was going to continue in the program, and asked the clinician to speak to the team about how to proceed. She also noted that her urges for self-injury were increasing as a result of this exchange.

It would have been easy (and likely more time efficient) for the clinician to send a quick email to the dietitian, to bring the issue to the next team meeting, or to walk down the hall and have a chat with a colleague about "what to do." However, none of these actions would have been effective for the client in the long term. The consultation-to-the-client approach means that we do not do for clients what they could reasonably learn to do for themselves. These experiences are viewed as opportunities to help our clients identify and describe emotions, activate the wise mind, and apply specific DBT skills to more effectively manage challenging situations. What occurs in the therapy context typically mirrors what happens outside of treatment, in this case a difficult interpersonal situation prompting escape behaviors and increasing urges for both ED and self-injurious behaviors. If clinicians jump in to solve problems for their clients, important learning opportunities are missed.

In this example, instead of talking to the dietitian on behalf of your client, you would use a collaborative stance and might do the following:

- Validate the difficulty of the situation
- Reinforce that your client felt comfortable sharing their experience with the RD
- Invite your client to practice a distress tolerance skill in session
- Work through the pros and cons of you speaking for your client versus your client approaching the situation themselves
- Practice wise-mind activation exercises
- Ask your client to write out a DEAR MAN script, a skill that teaches clients how to assertively ask for what they need while preserving the relationship and/or role-play how they might use this skill to bring their concerns back to the dietitian in an effective way.
- Reinforce the client's willingness to engage in these strategies and/or approach (versus avoid) the situation

When all members of the team observe this agreement, it creates opportunities to reinforce our clients when they are using skills. For instance, when your client approaches the dietitian to talk about their experience of the last meal planning session, the response of the dietitian (who supports the consultation-to-the-client agreement) might be: "I am so glad you are bringing your concerns to me directly. That isn't an easy thing to do. Can we talk more about how you felt judged and misunderstood by me because I definitely don't want you to feel that way?" Upholding the dialectical agreement, the dietitian recognizes that there are multiple truths operating (e.g., the dietitian felt she did understand the client, *and* the client felt judged and dismissed by the dietitian). Additionally, if the dietitian did, in fact, roll their eyes or express frustration in the session, the dietitian would own their behavior (fallibility agreement), validating how upsetting that would be, then offer a repair and work in partnership with the client to find ways to move forward.

However, it is important to acknowledge that there are times when the environment is discriminatory or marked by systemic barriers, abuse, and bias, as is often the case for our clients, given the preponderance of oppressive systems and the fat-phobic, pro-weight loss culture we live in. In these circumstances, you would take a more active approach and talk with your client about safety and whether there are ways to use the clinician's power and privilege to help.

## Consistency Agreement

In MED-DBT, we accept that treatment, and life, is full of inconsistencies. Different providers may offer differing advice, apply interventions in unique ways, or disagree about priorities. Our job is not to eliminate these contradictions but to help clients navigate them skillfully. Sayrs (2019) frames inconsistency not as a failure but as an opportunity for clients to practice coping with the unpredictability of the real world. Granato et al. (2022) remind us to critically examine how our definitions of consistency may be rooted in dominant culture and may unintentionally exclude other valid approaches.

Clients often encounter inconsistencies between therapist and dietitian, among external providers, or between personal and societal expectations. Rather than trying to reconcile every contradiction, we normalize this reality, validate the distress it causes, and teach clients to tolerate and respond to it effectively.

Clients often long for treatment environments that are predictable and consistent—particularly when the world around them has felt anything but. However, in both life and therapy, inconsistencies are inevitable. Sayrs (2019) notes that while DBT teams aim for clarity and cohesion, they also accept that "mix-ups are viewed as inevitable and isomorphic with the world we all live in." In other words, rather than trying to eliminate inconsistencies, DBT teaches us to treat them as opportunities for skill-building. Granato et al. (2022) extend this idea, reminding us to consider how dominant cultural norms shape our ideas of consistency and to remain open to perspectives that differ from our own.

A client might question why their doctor refused to run labs requested by the MED-DBT team or why they must follow a structured meal plan when friends skip meals without consequence. Others may feel confused when one clinician supports silence during meal exposures while another insists on verbal participation. These examples highlight common inconsistencies clients encounter—within treatment and in daily life.

Rather than shielding clients from these tensions, we prepare them for it. In our pretreatment orientation, we explain that different providers will have different roles, styles, and priorities. Not all will share the MED-DBT hierarchy of targets, and some may not be trained in DBT at all. We validate how difficult this can be, particularly for clients whose biology and history make them more sensitive to ambiguity. Then, we teach them how to navigate these situations skillfully, rather than resorting to symptom use.

Some ED clinicians worry that acknowledging inconsistency could be invalidating or even harmful. But within MED-DBT, we take a different stance: Your job is not to create a flawless or perfectly synchronized environment—it's to help your client survive and thrive in a world that isn't.

We work with clients to connect these experiences to real-life parallels: family members who undermine recovery, peers who celebrate disordered eating, or weight-normative systems that deny care based on BMI. We help them validate their pain *and* build a path forward, even when circumstances aren't fair or coherent. This fosters resilience—not through rigidity, but through radical acceptance and skillful action.

## Observing Limits Agreement

This agreement asks clinicians to openly acknowledge and respect their own limits—and those of others—without judgment. Limits are not signs of weakness; they are part of ethical, sustainable practice. By modeling this, we teach clients that it is safe and skillful to do the same. Sayrs (2019) encourages teams to observe their own limits and communicate them transparently. Granato et al. (2022) further suggest reflecting on how privilege may shape judgments about what constitutes a reasonable limit.

A therapist who feels overwhelmed by frequent crisis calls can use this agreement to reflect with their team and discuss boundaries with the client, not as rejection, but as collaboration. This opens the door for mutual understanding, emotional safety, and shared responsibility.

It is too often the case that we are not transparent with clients about our personal and professional limits. Depending on training models, some clinicians have been taught not to disclose personal limits while others report feeling uncomfortable discussing topics like burnout with clients so often avoid doing so. For example, a clinician attended a consultation team meeting and reported that they were having doubts about their ability to work with a client who was 3 months into treatment. The client was frequently medically unstable due to ongoing purging, exercise, and restricted eating. The team member reported that the client called for coaching multiple times per day to help with "feeling physically unwell" (e.g., dizziness, chest pain, extreme fatigue) but was not open to using skills. The clinician stated that the phone coaching calls felt more like supportive therapy and that they often lasted up to 30 minutes each time.

As the therapist spoke, she was visibly upset, and she questioned whether she was "cut out" to do this treatment. While the clinician had brought some of these issues to the consult team in prior weeks, the lack of progress in shaping the calls and the intensity of her burnout had not been named. The clinician also observed that she had not spoken directly with her client about what might increase her burnout as a preventative measure nor had they discussed how they would observe and describe limits over the course of therapy. While the clinician was trying to shape the calls, she was not letting the client know how they were impacting her motivation and sense of effectiveness. The clinician stated that her client had a long history of being "fired" by previous therapists, and she was afraid that giving any feedback about limits would be invalidating and would push the client away.

Limits are not unique to treatment; they are part of any healthy relationship. The observing limits agreement recognizes that treatment outcomes decline when limits are not clearly discussed, defined, and planned for. Without preparing for the ways we manage our limits, the chances of invalidation, burnout, and frustration increase for both therapist and client. We want to avoid letting things build up for weeks and months and then abruptly end treatment when the therapist or client reaches a breaking point. As a reflection exercise, first make a list of the things that might increase your feelings of burnout and/or ineffectiveness with your clients, then consider what gets in your way of talking about your limits with your clients.

There are all kinds of things that get in the way of therapists discussing their own limits. Some therapists feel that they "should" know how to handle challenging situations while others report feeling embarrassed to tell their team that they are struggling. Others avoid conflict or situations that might result in emotional intensity and end up fragilizing clients. Observing this agreement means that you are transparent with your clients about what might increase frustration or a sense of ineffectiveness (e.g., phone coaching calls about physical symptoms without willingness to try skills, arguing over whether bradycardia is a valid T1 behavior, slow meal plan changes). This is not intended to blame the patient, rather; to model that we all have limits and that talking about our limits at the start of treatment and throughout is a way to reduce challenges and work together more effectively.

But this isn't all about your limits! We elicit examples from our clients about what might burn *them* out (e.g., slow or no change in therapy, having to eat a meal without help in managing co-occurring suicidal thoughts, being told they cannot talk about self-injury or trauma in ED treatment). When you and your client nonjudgmentally observe limits, you are developing a way for client and therapist to co-create safe environments. We have found that these conversations are experienced as refreshing and unique to our clients who are not accustomed to having nonjudgmental and transparent conversations about limits. Most of the time, the people in their lives oscillate between not communicating limits or "walking on eggshells" and angrily conveying that a limit has been crossed. Such circumstances only lead to more emotional dysregulation, invalidation, and polarization in relationships.

## Phenomenological Empathy Agreement

> DBT team members agree, all other things being equal, to search for nonpejorative or phenomenologically empathic interpretations of clients' behavior.—Sayrs (2019, p. 9)

This agreement challenges us to assume the best in our clients, and in each other, even when the behaviors we're witnessing are confusing, frustrating, or intense. Rather than viewing clients through a judgmental lens, we strive to understand their behavior as logical responses to an unsettled biology and chronically invalidating environments. It also means holding space for our own emotional reactions while staying grounded in a non-pejorative framework.

As Sayrs (2019, p. 9) puts it, "DBT team members agree to hold one another nonjudgmentally in the DBT frame." In practice, this agreement plays out in how we talk about clients in team meetings, how we conceptualize challenges with engagement, and how we hold space for the impact of systemic forces—such as weight stigma or medical trauma—on our clients' behavior. In one consultation meeting, a team's frustration with a multidiagnostic client was palpable: eye rolls, exasperated sighs, and even a medical file labeled "BORDERLINE" in all caps. These reactions were understandable—this work is hard—but they were also a cue that the team had drifted from empathic understanding. We returned to the biosocial theory and treatment assumptions, not to shame the team, but to help them reconnect with the idea that even highly disruptive behavior is rooted in attempts to survive and self-regulate.

The phenomenological empathy agreement requires you to maintain a nonjudgmental and compassionate understanding of your client's behavior.

Your conceptualization of your client includes how culture, gender, body weight, diet culture, and other factors contribute to the patterns of behavior observed in treatment. Our clients have learned (and been reinforced) to use symptoms as methods of regulating an unsettled biology and managing invalidating environments. Instead of seeing a client as "borderline" or "losing weight to get attention," we instead accept that symptoms help clients to maintain a sense of stability, homeostasis, and predictability (in the short term). These behaviors are highly reinforced genetically and socially. When we struggle to find phenomenologically empathic views of a client, our team agrees to (1) validate how difficult this can be, (2) view their colleague through an empathic and nonjudgmental lens, (3) help the clinician explore what might be getting in the way, and (4) assist in returning to the biosocial theory to more compassionately conceptualize the client.

It is equally important to view the clinician/team through a phenomenologically empathic lens. Many practitioners are reinforced for thinking judgmentally about a client. We laugh with them, we roll our eyes in solidarity, people bond on teams by sharing in their frustration. We do not pass judgment on our colleagues, rather seek to facilitate change by supporting non-pejorative environments and views.

## Fallibility Agreement

This agreement is about owning our mistakes—without shame. In MED-DBT, we accept that we will inevitably drift from the model, misstep with clients, or act from bias. The key is to return, repair, and grow. Sayrs (2019) reminds us that fallibility is not a flaw—it is a given. Granato et al. (2022) build on this, highlighting the need to acknowledge privilege, power, and the inevitability of microaggressions in therapeutic relationships. Whether it's misgendering a client, underestimating the complexity of ARFID, or mishandling a session, we name it, repair it, and work to do better. Clients respond to this vulnerability with trust, and teams that practice fallibility consistently report greater cohesion, less burnout, and more authentic collaboration.

DBT teams, by nature, agree to be vulnerable. To be fallible is to accept that we make mistakes. As is true in any DBT model, MED-DBT accepts that no one is ever 100% reliable, effective, or flawless. We are going to judge, misunderstand, and drift from the therapy model. We are going to engage in therapy-interfering behaviors, microaggressions, and weight bias in spite of our ongoing efforts to do better. The organizations and systems we operate in are fallible. Healthcare itself is fallible. In having this conversation with a group of ED providers, several identified feeling afraid to make mistakes or acknowledge the ways in which they or their treatments were imperfect. As we continued to discuss this team agreement, many expressed relief: "It is so helpful to have space to be a real human in the room and use that as part of the therapy instead of feeling anxious and defensive when these things happen."

In working with many ED teams, we have used this agreement to address ways current treatments have been ill-equipped for those with ARFID, BED, and atypical anorexia. When clients report feeling invalidated and that their treatment needs have not been met, there is no need to be defensive. Rather, we acknowledge the truth in the client's perspective, which is that we have not done a sufficient job to build more diverse care pathways and that research and treatment are lacking in these areas. In working with one male client with ARFID, part of the pretreatment phase included the clinician discussing that he was still learning about this type of eating disorder and that he would likely make mistakes in how best to navigate the disorder along the way. This opened up a bigger discussion about fallibility in general and gave the client freedom to choose whether working with this particular clinician would be a good fit.

## Summary

The team agreements outlined in this chapter are not simply guidelines for professional conduct—they are living commitments that shape how we think, relate, and respond within the MED-DBT framework. By agreeing to uphold dialectics, observe our limits, practice fallibility, and view both clients and colleagues through an empathic, nonjudgmental lens, we create the kind of treatment environment that makes transformative work possible. These agreements help us stay aligned with the core DBT principles while meeting the complex needs of multidiagnostic ED clients with flexibility, humanity, and skill.

And yet, even with strong agreements in place, the work of understanding behavior doesn't stop there. In the next chapter, we explore how dialectical dilemmas—predictable patterns of extreme coping styles—emerge in response to the very biological vulnerabilities and invalidating environments we've already examined. Recognizing and naming these dilemmas is essential not only for deepening your case conceptualization but also for breaking through common treatment impasses with greater clarity and compassion.

# 7

# Dialectical Dilemmas in MED-DBT Treatment

In addition to formulating a solid and shared understanding of your client's experiences via the adapted biosocial theory, conceptualizing patterns of behavior through the perspective of dialectical dilemmas is a key therapeutic task. Dialectical dilemmas are patterns of coping that naturally and understandably occur as a result of living with particular biological vulnerabilities in the context of invalidating environments (Linehan, 1993). Transdiagnostic in nature, these coping responses have been categorized into pairs of seemingly opposite response styles (one extremely overcontrolled, the other extremely undercontrolled) that our clients vacillate between, hence the term "dialectical dilemma." While it is tempting to focus exclusively on ED (or other overt) symptoms, failure to address these underlying coping styles results in a lack of progress in treatment. Helping your client observe and describe dialectical dilemmas helps to do the following:

- Remove judgments and assumptions about why a behavior is happening (e.g., shifting from "My client is not motivated" to "This is a coping style")
- Increase self-compassion and reduce shame (e.g., shifting from "There's something wrong with me" to "I'm using a coping strategy that made sense at one point but may no longer be effective")
- Provide a more accurate understanding of where and why we get stuck in treatment
- Build more balanced ways of responding to emotions, relationships, and environments

## MED-DBT-Specific Dialectical Dilemmas

The original dialectical dilemmas, as outlined by Linehan (1993), describe predictable patterns of coping that emerge in individuals with high emotional sensitivity living within invalidating environments. The first, *emotion dysregulation versus self-invalidation,* captures the struggle between intense emotional experience and harsh internal self-criticism that arises when those emotions are not understood or supported. The second, *unrelenting crisis versus inhibited grieving,* describes a pattern where individuals either remain in constant turmoil or avoid processing distress altogether, unable to access the emotional space needed for resolution. The third, *active passivity versus apparent competence,* reflects the oscillation between relying heavily on others to solve problems and appearing outwardly capable while concealing internal distress. These dilemmas offer a powerful lens through which to understand behavior that might otherwise appear contradictory or treatment-interfering.

While this chapter focuses on the dialectical dilemmas our clients struggle with, it is equally important to acknowledge the role of *therapist imbalances,* a concept described in detail by Linehan (1993), to which the interested reader is directed for further exploration. We cannot do the topic justice here, but we also cannot ignore it. Without recognizing therapist imbalances, we risk focusing exclusively on one side of the dialectical paradigm. Therapists, like clients, can become polarized, rigid, or reactive in response to the intensity of the work. This is especially relevant in the treatment of EDs, where the pull of the medical model can create strong pressure to "rescue" the client, prioritize symptom elimination above all else, or override ambivalence in the name of safety. Consistent with Downs et al. (2025), polarization is not only a client phenomenon; it is embedded in the historical and systemic treatment of EDs. When clinicians fail to hold dialectical perspectives or default to singular "truths" about clients' experiences, epistemic invalidation occurs, further exacerbating client mistrust and disengagement. These imbalances, though well-intentioned, can lead to therapist behaviors that are overly controlling, emotionally distant, or, conversely, overly accommodating. In MED-DBT, we emphasize the transactional nature of the therapeutic relationship: Just as clients must navigate their own dialectical tensions, therapists must be equally mindful of their own. Remaining balanced, reflective, and dialectically flexible is not a luxury, it is essential to doing this work well.

Building on these foundational dilemmas, our clinical experience with multidiagnostic EDs has revealed additional, recurring tensions that are not fully captured by the original framework. In the sections that follow, we outline the MED-DBT-specific dialectical dilemmas that have emerged in our work; patterns that reflect the unique ways ED symptoms, emotional dysregulation, and treatment histories interact.

## Rigid, Overcontrolled Eating versus Absence of an Eating Plan

On one hand, our clients cling to a very inflexible, highly restrained, and oftentimes extremely compulsive style of eating. This can present as meticulous counting of calories or nutrients, only eating certain types of foods that are deemed "safe," eating only at specified times or in certain locations, ascribing to daily calorie limits, needing to cut foods into tiny pieces before consuming, restricting fluids, or compulsive exercise in order to get rid of calories or justify eating the next meal or snack. These behaviors are also related to your client's neurobiology (e.g., possible deficits in acetylcholine, metabolic differences that drive food choices/rules). Like the intense anxiety or anger a person with OCD might experience when blocked from completing a ritual, our clients feel extremely unsettled and emotionally dysregulated when unable to follow their rules and rituals around eating. Rigid, overcontrolled eating, as a coping style, is reinforced in several ways: it can soothe common psychological and physiological consequences of changing the rules ("If I change my eating, it will unbalance my macros and I can't deal with how that feels"); and in our diet-obsessed and fat-phobic world, controlled eating tends to be celebrated and viewed as a sign of health, control, and willpower.

At the other extreme is a style of coping defined by a complete letting go of any meal planning. Once bound by rules, you may be surprised to find that your client has abandoned anything and everything related to organizing and planning their food and fluid intake. Where they once operated in a meticulous fashion about when, where, and how much to eat, your client might now describe a pattern of chaotic and disorganized eating. They may describe uncertainty about how much they are eating and hold a belief that they are fine, that it is better not to plan for meals and snacks ("That was unhelpful anyway, right?"). Similar to the notion of "clean mind" in DBT-SUD (dialectical behavior therapy for substance use disorder), this extreme approach to meal planning (or the lack thereof) downplays the reality of how eating disorders are maintained. The short-term relief of forgoing rigid meal planning helps to reinforce this pattern of coping ("It was so time consuming to live that way, now I'm free") and others may experience them as more "fun" and flexible to be around. However, this sets our clients up for more intense and frequent ED behaviors alongside greater emotional distress in the long term. In our experience, poorly planned meals and snacks might give the illusion of a type of "ED freedom," but this usually increases the likelihood of restricted eating, binge eating, and other ED behaviors (Wisniewski & Kelly, 2003).

As a therapist, your job is to highlight this pattern when it arises and talk with your client about what makes sense about this coping style. There is validity in both extremes, *and* living in those extremes does not help our clients reach their life worth living goals. The goal is to help your client find a way to exist with food flexibly but with a plan. We want to help our clients develop skills so they are knowledgeable about where and when the next meal or snack will come from but not so compulsive that any deviation from the plan results in a crisis. We often talk about this as eating effectively. As the therapist, it will be necessary to monitor your own responses so as not to reinforce an unhelpful extreme. For example, a therapist who was very frustrated with the rigid eating habits of her client celebrated the client's abandonment of meal planning because it reduced her tension ("I don't have to deal with that anymore.") but did not address how the absence of a plan was causing a whole set of other problems. Our clients need to learn how to be both flexible and fluid with meal planning while being detailed and organized enough so as not to perpetuate the ED.

## Apparent Compliance versus Active Defiance

On one side of this dialectic, clients engage in behavior that gives the illusion of treatment compliance. They agree with you in session about using specific DBT skills to reduce purging, report following their meal plan, and may share examples of successful family meals or going to new restaurants. At first glance, this sounds wonderful, and it seems that treatment is moving along well. Except it isn't. You may find yourself asking why your client is still losing weight, why their ED thoughts are so intense, or why progress seems stalled given all the strategies being used. Upon further exploration, you uncover that your client has developed a way of coping that involves doing just enough to appear to be in agreement with treatment but not enough to create or sustain change. For example, your client says that he joined his friends for dinner at a new restaurant but, with further discussion, reports that he didn't actually eat anything while there. Or your client appears puzzled about weight loss because they are following their meal plan and not exercising, but, with exploration, you learn that she is eating low-calorie products, no added fats, and is walking 5 kilometers to and from work each day.

Apparent compliance can also present as the client demanding time and attention from the provider ("I am here and want treatment") but only on the client's terms (e.g., "But I can't be here every week or attend skills groups or work on staying alive"). These behaviors tend to be confusing for practitioners and families because it seems like the individual is hard at work and in agreement with the treatment plan, yet things keep falling apart. The difficulty is that appearing compliant often works! For example, your client may learn that apparently compliant behavior distracts people (therapist, family, friends, teacher, or coach) from focusing on ED behaviors. In their article on this topic, Wisniewski and Ben-Porath (2015) share the example of a patient whose mother asked her if she ordered pizza at a friend's house; the patient says yes and her mother's anxiety is alleviated. However, if the mother had asked more questions, she may have discovered that her daughter didn't actually *eat* any of the pizza. The apparently compliant behavior has distracted and the patient is not blocked from or punished for ED behaviors.

Paradoxically, your clients oscillate between appearing compliant and actively defying treatment. Traditional ED treatment programs are rule-bound by design. Patients attending ED treatments generally receive a prescription regarding what, when, and how much they can eat, drink, and move, while at the same time other behaviors, such as excessive cutting of food or use of condiments are proscribed (i.e., prohibited). The prescriptive and proscriptive model employed in traditional ED programs is effective for many, but not all, ED patients. Specifically, the prescriptions typically encountered in ED treatment (e.g., "You must . . . ") can be experienced as invalidating ("You don't get how hard this is to eat") and, as such, result in refusing or rebelling against treatment providers ("You can't make me . . . "). The typical proscriptions (e.g., "You cannot . . . ") result in similar responses ("I will . . . and you can't stop me!"). These reactive responses to being told what to do may cause clients to be discharged from treatment prematurely, be seen by providers and loved ones as signs of "not wanting to get better," and be those that negatively impact the therapeutic relationship. Over time, our clients learn that actively defiant behaviors may prompt individuals to decrease expected/desired change from them.

The back-and-forth between appearing compliant and actively defying treatment can be confusing and unsettling for clinicians, families, and clients. As emphasized by Wisniewski and Ben-Porath (2015), conceptualizing these behaviors as a dialectical dilemma is very important; otherwise, the risk of viewing the client's behavior as "resistant" or "manipulative" persists. In MED-DBT, we see this style of coping as a natural and predictable outcome rooted in a client's biotemperament and as a result of experiencing invalidating or ineffective environments. The goal is to resolve the dilemma by finding more balanced ways of approaching the distress of treatment. This may mean increasing honesty or decreasing "keeping secrets," increasing dialectical thinking in treatment, increasing ability to name emotions, increasing distress tolerance skills, orienting to radical acceptance, and using GIVE skills for effective communication. The GIVE skills are designed to help individuals maintain healthy relationships and build connection during interpersonal interactions. GIVE stands for *G*entle, *I*nterested, *V*alidate, and *E*asy manner. These skills support the goal of keeping the relationship intact while asserting one's needs or setting boundaries. GIVE is particularly useful in emotionally charged situations, helping clients stay grounded and effective without escalating conflict or damaging the relationship.

## Expecting Independence versus Fostering Dependence

Rathus and Miller (2000) introduced a number of dialectical dilemmas specific to their work with adolescents and families. One of those dilemmas was "forcing autonomy versus fostering dependence" in the parent–child relationship. When it comes to ED treatment, we observe a similar dilemma related to food, weight, shape, and recovery. On one hand, treatment providers (and families) may expect a level of independence around making food choices, going grocery shopping ("When are they going to do this themselves?"), eating meals and snacks ("They should be able to eat more on their feared food list"), being weighed ("Why are they still so upset by this?"), and tolerating physical changes ("It is important for them to sit with discomfort"). Providers/families can quickly grow frustrated at what is perceived as a lack of progress in the domain of independence ("Why are they not moving from Stage 1 to Stage 2 treatment?"). This is a significant dilemma for our clients who also long for independence, but in traditional ED treatments are often not provided the skills to achieve that goal.

Simultaneously, the environment may act in ways that encourage dependence. This may include providers or families doing all of the meal planning for the client, treating clients as fragile during meals (e.g., "this is too hard for you to learn to manage on your own"), talking for the client at medical appointments, scheduling meetings for the client instead of teaching the client to coordinate appointments themselves, or treating a client as incapable of making decisions or contributing to discussions about their treatment.

It is important as a therapist to stay mindful of times when you might reinforce either end of this dilemma, as well as to notice, with your client, when they are caught moving between these two poles. We help our clients resolve this pattern by teaching them the skills they need to master more independence. We use the consultation-to-the-client approach to teach and shape their ability to act for themselves (e.g., having them call the physician for an appointment). We orient and role-play how to use DEAR MAN skills around an upcoming food outing with family or to ask for a medication change at their next physician's appointment so they can learn to be more independent skillfully. At the same time, we recognize that learning these skills in the context of an eating disorder and in the presence of additional co-occurring conditions takes time. Too much independence is likely to backfire. Fostering dependence is also not a long-term solution. Our clients need structure, rules at times, and guidance—and they need opportunities to learn to handle food, eating, body image, emotions, and relationships on their own.

## Normalizing Pathological Behaviors versus Pathologizing Normative Behaviors

Another dialectical dilemma from the adolescent model has important relevance in MED-DBT. Just as Rathus and Miller (2000) observed an oscillation within their adolescent clients between pathologizing normal teenage behavior (e.g., experimentation with marijuana) and minimizing pathological behavior (e.g., selling drugs at school), we recognize a similar dilemma in our clients. When applied to our work, the heart of this dilemma is the ability to differentiate developmentally and culturally normative behavior around food, body, and health from behavior that may be appropriate but causes significant harm and/or substantially reduces quality of life.

On one end of the dialectic, your clients may adamantly uphold the position that they are fine even in the presence of disconfirming data ("I am an athlete so a heart rate in the 40s is normal"), that their ED symptoms are not concerning ("My health is fine because my labs are stable"), or view dieting as part of a healthy lifestyle ("Intermittent fasting is normal and prescribed by my doctor so it is fine for me"). In one case, our client, a physician who would run miles per day on fractured bones, argued that her behavior was normal and "just the life of a runner." Perhaps this is the ultimate internalization of the invalidating environment in which the whole of diet culture is accepted as normative. It is also possible that this behavior reflects anosognosia, the brain's inability to recognize its own illness, compounded by the effects of malnourishment on self-perception. In either case, it presents a challenge when trying to elicit change.

We also have to remember that our clients are not the only ones who might normalize harmful behaviors. Family members may ignore ED behaviors ("She has so much self-control!"). Similarly, practitioners or families can become so desensitized to high-risk behaviors that dangerous symptoms or circumstances are overlooked or perceived as less harmful than other client behaviors (e.g., accepting daily purging because the client is no longer suicidal).

At the other end of the dialectic, your clients (and their families or treatment providers) may pathologize normative behaviors. This is usually observed as an overreaction or attempt to discourage behaviors that would be considered developmentally and culturally appropriate. This can be a very challenging task in the ED space, particularly when so many normative behaviors can be hard to distinguish from ED symptoms. For example, in North America, it is statistically normal (as in "what people do" vs. "This is a 'good thing' to do") to want to lose weight or change one's appearance in a weight-obsessed world. It is normal to want body autonomy, to be in control of what foods one eats, or to look for a sense of safety in one's body.

For parents and practitioners who have witnessed life-threatening behaviors and the tenacious nature of an ED, the presentation of normative desires or behaviors can be excessively feared and controlled. One parent of a transitional-age youth described taking away their loved one's internet access and vehicle when they expressed having a "bad body image day" 6 months into recovery. Understandably, an admission of body loathing was scary for this parent, who remembered all the times such statements meant the start of a long and painful relapse. However, having "bad body image days" is part of an expected and normative experience that we want our clients to work with. A therapist described his view about his client's request to not be weighed in later stages of treatment as a sure sign that they were not well and in need of more intensive treatment. While there are important times when weighing a client is necessary, a desire for body autonomy is not an inappropriate request.

Relatedly, your client may find themselves confused about what is normative and may actively label common experiences as abnormal. One client described herself as a treatment failure because she still felt nervous wearing a bathing suit at the beach. Another client who was doing a great job for many months with her eating pathologized any deviation from her meal plan as signs that she was relapsing. Another example is the person who has been taught that leaving food on their plate is restriction (pathological) who may struggle once they learn to pay attention to hunger and fullness cues and wonder about leaving food on their plate (normal if you are full and don't have an ED). While some of these may be indicators of a worsening presentation or lack of progress, they are also normative behaviors in Western culture.

Ultimately, we want to help our clients and their therapists find a middle ground between ignoring dangerous and harmful behaviors and censoring or pathologizing behaviors that are expected and normative. We can do this by providing psychoeducation about what is normal (statistically and developmentally) when it comes to bodies, eating, and working through ED treatment. Highlighting how much we *don't* know in some of these areas is also helpful in order to steer away from nondialectical thinking (e.g., "there is only one way to look at this behavior"). Help your client observe and describe when they judge, criticize, or "should" themselves for experiencing what is to be expected. For some clients, this may mean radically accepting that others may hold very different beliefs when it comes to normative behaviors when there is a history of illness severity. We also want to help our clients take dangerous and harmful behavior seriously. We do this by nonjudgmentally acknowledging when this behavior happens, exploring how avoiding harmful behaviors may be reinforced or otherwise functional, teaching your client how to evaluate risk appropriately, and developing ways to activate wise mind in these situations.

## Summary

Dialectical dilemmas are naturally occurring coping styles that develop as a result of the interaction between biotemperament and the invalidating environment. Clients vacillate between extremes in an effort to regulate their emotions, thoughts, physical feelings, and relationships. Your client may exhibit one or more of these dilemmas but is certainly not expected to have all of them. Your job is to observe these transdiagnostic patterns with your client, teach them about their development and functionality, explore how the patterns help/hinder the path toward a life worth living, and work collaboratively to integrate skills to modify these patterns. Understanding your client's dialectical dilemmas lays the foundation for effective treatment—but before the formal work of MED-DBT can begin, there must be a shared commitment to the process. The next chapter outlines the essential pretreatment phase, where motivation is strengthened, expectations are clarified, and both therapist and client prepare for the challenges and demands of the work ahead.

# Part III
# Getting Ready for Treatment

This part of the book focuses on preparing both you and your client for the work of comprehensive MED-DBT. Before treatment can begin, you'll need to establish shared goals, clarify the structure of the program, and assess your client's willingness and capacity to engage in the treatment process. These chapters walk you through the essential components of the pretreatment phase, including how to facilitate the life worth living discussion and how to collaboratively establish a treatment hierarchy that aligns with your client's needs and values. By the end of this section, you will have the tools to set the foundation for a clear, focused, and commitment-based start to therapy.

This part of the book includes the following:

- Chapter 8: Laying the Foundation: Early Steps in the MED-DBT Pretreatment Phase
- Chapter 9: Strengthening Commitment: Later Tasks in MED-DBT Pretreatment
- Chapter 10: The Life Worth Living Discussion
- Chapter 11: What to Target and When

# 8

# Laying the Foundation

## Early Steps in the MED-DBT Pretreatment Phase

The pretreatment phase of MED-DBT is a deliberate and essential stage that lays the groundwork for all subsequent treatment. In this chapter, we provide an overview of the rationale for this phase, outlining the structure of the four pretreatment sessions and their critical clinical aims. This includes identifying and addressing common obstacles to engagement, assessing medical stability, and initiating conversations around the willingness to stay alive. Given the complexity of multidiagnostic EDs, these sessions are not merely about readiness, they are about ensuring that the conditions for treatment to be safe, collaborative, and effective are in place. You'll learn how to hold the dialectic between urgency and pacing, between safety and autonomy, and how to stay anchored when clients are unsure, withdrawn, or ambivalent. This chapter equips you to begin the pretreatment phase with clarity and intention, while setting up the deeper collaborative work that follows.

## Overview and Rationale

If your client has been assessed and deemed a good fit for MED-DBT, the next step in the process is the pretreatment phase, often referred to as the motivation and commitment phase. This phase of treatment is delivered in a four-session format designed to ensure that our clients are clear about what treatment involves. In DBT, we do not assume that treatment begins just because someone is sitting across from us stating that they want help. As we do in standard DBT, MED-DBT does not actually "start" until the pretreatment phase is complete. Why is this? Linehan (1993) developed the model to include motivation and commitment work at the outset in order to target the significant uncertainty and ambivalence our clients experience. People want to feel better, *and* it requires a lot of work. The pretreatment phase is particularly important as it lays the groundwork for that inevitable time in the future when your client says, "This is too hard," and is not sure they want to continue working on these issues. By working through the pretreatment phase, you will already have had these conversations and will link back to them many times over the course of treatment.

The pretreatment phase is also highly relevant to our work, where ambivalence and differences with respect to degrees of insight around illness severity (e.g., anosognosia) are common for our clients. Individuals living with multidiagnostic ED presentations struggle with sustaining motivation due to illness complexity, pervasive invalidation (sometimes from the mental health field), and histories of repeated, unsuccessful attempts with treatment. Moreover, many clients describe traditional ED systems of care as ineffective for their unique needs. Reasons for this include disagreement with theoretical models, feeling unheard or lacking collaboration with providers, experiencing stigma and judgment when they were unable to make required changes, a lack of acceptance-based or harm reduction approaches, and engaging with systems that do not provide support for other co-occurring and related symptoms (e.g., suicide, self-injury, neurodiversity; Asaria, 2025). By the time they reach us, many individuals feel burnt out with treatment or describe wariness about "trying again" for fear of the same approaches being applied.

As described earlier, standard ED treatments are predominantly change-focused. CBT-ED, FBT, as well as higher levels of care require patients to engage in mechanical eating (i.e., following a meal plan and eating at prescribed intervals), weight and food monitoring, and cognitive modification in the very beginning of the intervention. If treatment engagement is not observed in these early stages, the data demonstrate poor outcomes. In response to this, ED therapists commonly describe feeling the need to move clients quickly into action, are fearful of the medical risks if change does not occur swiftly, and do not feel comfortable with interventions that are perceived as "slowing down" movement.

On the other hand, lack of treatment engagement also typically results in early discharge from traditional ED treatments. In one setting in which we provided training and consultation, the team reported that they felt the need to "fix, fix, fix," and that any "resistance" or lack of patient engagement prompted an increase in change strategies; this is especially true for clients of low body weight or where medical stability may be an issue. MED-DBT may be a viable option for those clients who have not been helped by evidence-based treatments since they more directly address both acceptance and change.

While moving quickly and wanting to help a client stabilize their health and eating makes sense, the push for change in the absence of acceptance-based strategies tends to slow down motivation and commitment for our clients and can increase invalidation. Models that are heavily change-focused are problematic as many clients do not arrive to treatment in a state of readiness to change, or may be willing to focus on reducing some symptoms (e.g., self-injury, substance use, family tensions) but not others (e.g., restricting, purging, exercise). Clients may also agree to anything because they are in a crisis and when the crisis begins to resolve, ambivalence arises. Our clients tend to be in *precontemplative* or *contemplative* stages of change, which standard treatments are not equipped to manage.

This mismatch between the needs of our clients and traditional ED approaches (active stage of change) has resulted in assumptions that our clients are not motivated to change or are "difficult to treat." In our view, this is not the case at all. Our experience is that our clients are quite motivated to reduce suffering and want a more stable and satisfying life, and they require a different space and approach in order to feel safe and supported enough to pursue those goals. For example, our clients often experience early change-based approaches as invalidating or threatening. The "ask" of traditional therapies (e.g., to eat regularly, get on a scale, eat feared foods, challenge ED thoughts) seems impossible and reductionist. For individuals who have difficulty regulating emotion, are neurodivergent, have trauma histories, struggle with co-occurring illnesses, and have been invalidated by the system itself, requiring such change can feel as though providers simply do not understand the intersecting sensory, perceptual, traumatic, and sociocultural factors and identities at play.

Clients commonly report that past treatments have expected them to make changes without the scaffolding of support in areas such as self-regulation and management of pervasive invalidation, leaving them feeling exposed and more vulnerable. Approaches that are predominantly change-focused also reinforce the notion that harm reduction and acceptance-based models are not useful nor in line with mainstream definitions of effective treatment and recovery. Our clients don't agree with these formulations and assumptions, nor do we. Traditional therapies can be conceptualized as more black and white in terms of processes, flow, and treatment expectations, whereas our clients need something more dialectical. MED-DBT acknowledges that pushing for change as a primary stance guarantees an overactive threat system, an increase in emotion dysregulation, and a decrease in the client's ability to trust, engage, and take in new information. Our clients are willing to make changes, albeit more slowly than most programs are comfortable with; it is necessary to meet them where they are at, at least to start. This need to move slowly is not true for all clients with EDs but is often the case for our clients.

## Potential Challenges

As you read this chapter and those that follow, you will note that the way we engage with our clients is quite different both in terms of style and with respect to how we conceptualize and formulate goals. For those trained in standard DBT, you will be comfortable with the nature of pretreatment, the use of commitment strategies, and the dialectical nature of our conversations. We imagine, however, that you will be less familiar with how to engage clients around medical stability, food and fluid intake, and working with the ancillary medical team. Your knowledge and direct attention to weight science and the nuances of ED experiences are necessary as you work through this treatment phase. It may also be challenging to know what limits to observe or how to orient clients to contingency protocols related to EDs.

For those trained in ED approaches, you will be fluent with ED psychoeducation and recognize some of our strategies from motivational interviewing approaches that have been applied to EDs in the past. We imagine this phase will be a departure from how you typically begin working with clients. The way we target eating, body weight, and medical stability will be different. The pretreatment phase can feel slow to traditionally trained ED clinicians and/or like it collides with traditional approaches or system pressures to treat quickly.

The other confounding factor is that many patients with EDs are referred to higher levels of care at the outset of treatment or told that higher levels of care will be required if quick change is not met. As discussed in Chapter 2, it is also true that many ED practitioners do not give clients the option of outpatient treatment and require that they be seen from the start in a higher level of care. Our experience, however, has been the opposite. We observe that working with these early treatment "blocks'" through an adherent pretreatment phase is predictive of a positive outcome. Keep in mind that, despite being referred to as "pretreatment," this is a potent phase of the model when applied thoroughly.

## Goals of the Pretreatment Phase

Importantly, during this phase, your client is not yet "in" the MED-DBT program. There is no agreement yet that you and your client will work together. Unlike other treatments in which a client can reasonably assume that the first session marks the beginning of a longer-term relationship, the pretreatment phase in MED-DBT may or may not lead to admission to the comprehensive program. The purpose of this stage is for you and your client to explore feasibility, life worth living goals, pros and cons of using this approach, and whether committing to the program makes sense at this time. Notably, you are not yet considered to be providing active therapy to your client. Skills groups, phone coaching, meal planning, weighing, and medical/crisis management are not offered during the pretreatment phase. This can feel very uncomfortable for traditionally trained ED practitioners who are used to case managing and moving quickly, especially in the face of instability. The purpose of this phase is to determine if your client is able to participate in the comprehensive program and whether you can increase willingness and/or reduce early obstacles that will interfere with receiving care. Thus, your client is free to see other providers while these sessions are held and is encouraged to maintain any existing support until a decision is made.

The pretreatment phase is a distinct and time-limited process that follows the assessment and is designed to be highly collaborative. As stated, the tasks and approaches used in this treatment phase are typically different from what clients (and clinicians) have experienced in previous ED approaches; therefore, it is important to orient new clients to the goals, tasks, and duration of this process. Transparency about the process and goals of this phase is an important element of commitment work. You may want to consider creating handouts for your clients to supplement the details of this phase of treatment. With this in mind, the first four sessions are organized around the following tasks:

- Building a working alliance and enhancing commitment to treatment
- Cultivating willingness to stay alive in terms of both suicide and the ED
- Identifying life worth living goals

- Developing a collaborative conceptualization of the client's current problems using the MED-DBT biosocial theory
- Orienting to the modes, assumptions, and interventions used in MED-DBT
- Discussing potential obstacles to the treatment
- Making a decision and completing paperwork

The pretreatment phase involves an average of four consecutive, weekly sessions with a MED-DBT trained clinician. Certainly, each client is different and additional sessions may be required to work through the material. That said, it is important not to prolong the pretreatment phase or begin to provide active treatment before it is complete. A clear end date is recommended. If your client is missing sessions, this is addressed right away as treatment-interfering. We point out to clients that pretreatment can't be effective if they are not present or if this phase takes too long. At the same time, it is important not to rush this phase.

Sometimes clients attend pretreatment saying they are willing and able to do anything and are eager to start group and phone coaching. We have had clinicians report to us that a client is ready after two pretreatment sessions. While it can be tempting to move forward with that kind of motivation, we advise against it. It is important that potential clients have time to hear all of the information about how the program operates, work through examples of how MED-DBT would approach their unique symptoms and goals, and take time between each pretreatment session to review and think about the information provided before making a decision. Rushing in without agreement tends to perpetuate burnout and hopelessness for clients when things don't work out, yet again.

## Case Study: Lia

Lia was a 34-year-old female client who attended an initial therapy session with a student therapist who was newer to MED-DBT. Lia began the pretreatment phase after 4 months on the clinic's waiting list. She presented with hypokalemia, purging multiple times per day, excessive physical activity (4+ hours per day), and frequent suicidal ideation and self-injurious behavior. After the first pretreatment session, Lia called the office four times asking to speak to the MED-DBT clinician about her symptoms. The therapist advised the admin team to reiterate to Lia the nature of their relationship during this phase of treatment, to tell her that if she was worried about her health to seek medical care, and that she would see her at the next scheduled session. On the fifth call, Lia reported that she was suicidal. The therapist, feeling anxious, called Lia right away to problem-solve. The next day, Lia called the admin office three times requesting to talk to the therapist. Again, the admin team advised that this was not available during pretreatment and for Lia to use crisis lines or seek urgent care at the hospital. She then left a fourth message stating she was not going to do MED-DBT. The therapist emailed Lia to offer soothing and to reiterate that she would hopefully see her at the next scheduled session. Lia thanked the therapist but sent four other long emails to her in the days that followed.

Lia attended the second session. The therapist taught biosocial theory, which Lia felt was helpful. Again, the therapist reoriented Lia to the rationale for the pretreatment phase and agreed with her that waiting was hard when desperately needing help. They developed a crisis plan to manage the time between appointments. Two days after this session, the therapist received a call from Lia's physician stating that Lia had been admitted to the hospital for chest pains and low potassium. The physician wondered why treatment hadn't started yet and emphasized that Lia should be in a skills group immediately after discharge from the hospital. The therapist reported feeling anxious and pressured and asked the team if an exception could be made to rush this client into a skills group and to start phone coaching right away. The team helped the therapist maintain the limits that guide the nature of pretreatment.

When Lia was released from the hospital, she missed her scheduled appointment but called the office three times that same day because she was suicidal and needed to talk to the therapist. The therapist set up an emergency session that day with the client. Over the next three weeks, the therapist and client continued to spend time managing crises but did not cover the pretreatment material. They oscillated between psychoeducation and support, and at the end of seven weeks Lia was no further along in her stability or commitment and was feeling upset with the team that more wasn't being done. The therapist had grown anxious and frustrated. Lia's physician called again and the client's family, also frustrated, demanded to know why they had "wasted so much time and money when nothing had been done."

In MED-DBT, the importance of medical and nutritional stability is of paramount importance; however, the manner in which we engage with clients around these targets is quite different. While the therapist's intent was to help, rushing into active treatment often backfires for our clients. Instead, in MED-DBT, this tension is used right away to highlight the concept of dialectics: the client desperately needs help now *and* still must complete four weeks of pretreatment before entering the comprehensive model. The stance of the therapist is one of pining for the client ("I really hope we can work together") while observing limits ("And, if this has a shot of working, we need time to talk about what is actually involved in this model so you can decide if it makes sense for you"). During this stage of the treatment, the focus is on orienting to the model and enhancing commitment without jumping in to solve the problems or provide treatment prematurely. The nature of this tension highlights one of the central functions of the MED-DBT consult team: aiding clinicians to work through high-stress and high-risk behaviors and their own emotion regulation in order to stay adherent to the model and make wise-mind treatment decisions.

## Building a Working Alliance and Enhancing Motivation

A key function of this phase is to establish a connection with your client and to increase willingness to work together. This is accomplished in several ways. Your stance, which is grounded in assumptions about clients and MED-DBT treatment assumptions (see Chapter 5), establishes a safe and validating space for our clients to discuss their concerns and to learn about MED-DBT. Throughout treatment, and especially during the pretreatment phase, your fluency with DBT commitment and stylistic strategies is essential to adherent delivery (see Linehan, 1993; Swenson, 2016). We value the lived experience of our clients, work to reduce power dynamics, and operate as co-creators in terms of making sense of our clients' problems and developing a feasible treatment plan. With our knowledge that clients have endured chronic invalidation both in terms of their biotemperament and their eating, weight, and shape (in addition to other possible forms of traumatic invalidation; Harned, 2022; Linehan, 1993), we aim to establish a space that is weight-inclusive, gender-affirming, dialectical, validating, and nonjudgmental.

Whether the client decides to pursue the MED-DBT program or not, this phase is a powerful intervention in its own right. Your client enters into a space in which they are heard, seen, and valued while learning about MED-DBT and its potential suitability. If your client only completed the pretreatment phase and decided against MED-DBT, the intention is that they would have had a positive experience engaging with you and walk away with a solid conceptualization or "road map" for why the journey has been so challenging to date and what options they have moving forward. Notice, though, that for the commitment phase to work, you must be willing to let your client go!

## Cultivating Willingness to Stay Alive: Addressing Suicide and Life-Threatening ED Behaviors

In standard DBT, your client must be willing to target suicidal and self-injurious behaviors—in other words, they must be willing to stay alive. This has unique and specific relevance to those with EDs that go beyond typical DBT targets. For those with EDs, the risk of death is elevated. According to Deloitte Access Economics (2020), one person dies every 52 minutes as a direct result of their eating disorder. Starvation, weight cycling, purging, laxative abuse, excessive exercise, and more cause widespread damage to the brain and the body that can lead to sudden cardiac failure and other imminently life-threatening conditions. Given that your client needs to stay alive in order to have enough time to see if this treatment can work, we need to determine whether our clients are willing to address suicide *and* imminently life-threatening ED behaviors.

Importantly, at this stage of treatment, the frame is not about setting goals to achieve a full ED recovery. Instead, the goal is to determine whether your client is willing to stay stable enough in treatment to not die from their ED. This distinction between staying alive (i.e., willingness to increase food intake to resolve bradycardia) versus committing to full ED recovery (i.e., willingness to follow a full meal plan, stop exercising, and reach a certain target weight) is an important one. Of course, if someone *wants* and is *ready* to commit to full recovery, we will embrace this. However, for others it is like asking someone to commit to running a marathon when their only physical activity for the past year has been to walk around the block.

### Is Your Client Willing to Do What Is Needed to Stay Alive during Pretreatment?

For many of our clients, discussions about medical stability have been difficult. They are expected to be medically stable to access outpatient programming or are quickly referred to higher levels of care. Our clients have often been labeled as unwilling or not motivated enough to maintain stability and have been said to "prefer the sick role" when usual ED interventions have not resulted in change. We have a different view of what is happening with our clients. We do not assume that our clients want to be unwell or live a life in and out of the hospital. While it may be true that they have been reinforced at times when unwell (e.g., receiving more care or compassion when medically unstable), we do not believe that our clients want to die or feel desperately unwell. Our clients don't have control over the ED itself, *but* they have control over making changes in their behaviors that will allow them to remain medically stable. We maintain a dialectical stance as we have these discussions, observing that the client may not have the skills to maintain medical stability and yet we have the confidence and expectation that this is something they can achieve. As we discuss the rationale for staying alive (Target I), we do so with the intention of collaborating on how to work together to resolve obstacles. At this stage, the client does not have to agree to stay alive forever, just to work on stability in order to try pretreatment. You can build motivation to stay alive for a longer period of time later on.

It has been our experience that practitioners working with MED clients have used the "you are going to die from this illness" card as a way to scare the client into better behavior. If they are sitting in your office, this intervention likely has not worked. We can't tell you the number of clients who have said: "they said that my low potassium was going to kill me, but here I am . . ." Your job as the therapist is to help your client figure out the line between ignoring or not believing that they are impacted by the ED versus the idea that they could die at any moment (likely not valid).

## Collaboratively Collect Data to Determine Stability

Beginning in pretreatment (and potentially at various stages in the program), clients are asked to provide up-to-date (e.g., within the last 10–14 days) vitals and lab work to aid in the determination of medical stability. We cannot tell by looking at someone if they are physically stable. In addition, many of our clients have interoceptive awareness (and other sensory/perceptual) difficulties and/or have high physical tolerance levels such that they are less attuned to their own medical conditions. Obtaining current labs/vitals provides an objective assessment of what is going on inside the body. While clients may not know how to manage medical stability right away, their willingness to get labs done is in keeping with the notion of "doing everything you can to stay alive." We also discuss the client's history of instability in order to establish the hierarchy. For example, at what weight/level of behaviors have they become unstable in the past? If your client historically becomes unstable at 115 pounds, weight loss approaching this value would be targeted as therapy-interfering. For more information on international guidelines on medical testing in eating disorders, see the Academy for Eating Disorders (2021).

While getting lab work done may seem like a fairly straightforward request, it often isn't. Many clients have been invalidated or felt unsafe when discussing eating disorders or body weight with medical providers. Clients report being subjected to weight stigma and bias, having requests for medical monitoring be dismissed, and/or being told that they are not "sick enough" to warrant lab work. During the pretreatment phase, we have had physicians refuse to order labs/vitals, dismiss low heart rates (e.g., 38 beats/minute) as signs of "athleticism," or question why a client in a larger body even requires such evaluation. These experiences underscore the need to refrain from making assumptions about why clients have not been able to access medical tests. Avoiding medical providers might have a protective function!

While some clients are able to get labs and vitals done in time for the first appointment, others need the first session with a MED-DBT therapist to discuss the rationale for the medical stability criteria and work on reducing obstacles to obtaining the necessary tests. If clients do not have lab work at the first pretreatment session, the therapist assesses for obstacles, helps with problem solving, and requests the data before the next scheduled session. It is essential to validate and maintain a compassionate position while pushing for change. While we emphasize the consultation-to-the-client approach (in which we help the client act skillfully on their own, rather than intervening for the client), it may be necessary to act on behalf of your client if their medical providers are unwilling to provide the necessary testing. In our experience, it is more effective to put this request in writing, rather than leaving a voice message or contacting a medical office via telephone. Written requests become part of the patient's medical file and are harder to dismiss. As discussed in Chapter 6, efforts to get a physician on your team are recommended. We find many doctors and family health teams are eager to have experts to collaborate with when it comes to ED care.

In contrast, clinicians sometimes worry that they are not equipped to use lab test data, as most are not medical providers. The collection of these data does not require therapists to interpret the findings. Lab and vitals need to be conducted and interpreted by a qualified medical provider (e.g., physician, nurse, nurse practitioner). The results that the therapist receives (e.g., bloodwork results, ECG results) have already been interpreted by the physician or cardiologist. The therapist simply reviews and discusses them with the client, and helps the client to problem-solve how to get more information when needed and/or consult with their physician about how to treat any instability.

## Medical Stability versus Instability in Pretreatment

If your client is medically stable in pretreatment, provide reinforcement, educate on medical instability and risks in EDs, and discuss whether your client is willing to continue to maintain medical stability during treatment. Always keep in mind your client's history of medical instability. Discuss that if symptoms worsen (e.g., weight loss, chest pain, dizziness, increased purging) or if certain behaviors that have historically been connected with instability arise, we would need to get updated labs and vitals right away. Medical stability is an ongoing target, just as one would monitor for suicide and self-injury in standard DBT.

If your client is medically unstable in pretreatment, reinforce that they said they were willing to get lab work done (this demonstrates commitment toward staying alive), continue to educate on medical instability and risks in EDs, discuss the pros and cons of staying alive with respect to doing MED-DBT (i.e., we can't be successful if you are dead), and use DBT commitment strategies to enhance readiness and willingness to resolve medical instability. The following example demonstrates some of these strategies with a client who is purging and has hypokalemia. Make note of when and how the therapist uses commitment (freedom to choose) and stylistic strategies (consultation-to-the-client, irreverence, dialectics, observing limits).

*Therapist*: Thank you for getting the bloodwork and vitals to me so quickly. I appreciate that.

*Client*: Well, you said I had to have it.

*Therapist*: Yes, I did ask you to do this. I appreciate it (therapist looks at lab results and reviews out loud). I notice here that your potassium is flagged as low?

*Client*: Yeah, that always happens. It's fine.

*Therapist*: Okay, so this is something you've seen before?

*Client*: Yup.

*Therapist*: You don't seem so concerned by it . . . (therapist pauses) and I am noticing my own concern as I look at this.

*Client*: (*rolling his eyes*) It's fine, really.

*Therapist*: You sound a bit frustrated. I wonder if I can clarify with you what I am thinking? [seeking agreement to talk further rather than just assuming they are interested in your perspective]

*Client*: Sure.

*Therapist*: Okay, thanks. So, like we were talking about last session, some eating disorder symptoms are associated with higher rates of death. One of the factors that contribute to those rates are things like electrolyte imbalances, low potassium being one of them. It is a condition known as hypokalemia. Have you heard of this before?

*Client*: Yeah, my electrolytes have been off in the past and when I was an inpatient they had to monitor me every few days for a while.

*Therapist*: What was that like for you?

*Client*: I hated it! So stupid. I don't think I am really that sick.

*Therapist*: It can definitely be frustrating to have to get labs done often, especially if you don't agree with the rationale.

*Client*: Exactly!

*Therapist*: I think this is a good conversation for us to be having because, as far as I know, treatment can't work if you are dead. [irreverent communication]

*Client*: (*Gives a little laugh.*) Well . . . obviously!

*Therapist*: (*Smiles back.*) So we agree on that?

*Client*: I get what you mean, but I am not going to die. I haven't died yet!

*Therapist*: I'm glad you haven't died yet. [reinforcement] So we agree that people who are dead don't do well in treatment. The question seems to be whether we agree on what is *imminently* life-threatening. Sounds like right now, you don't believe you are sick enough or in need of that much medical observation.

*Client*: I just don't think my electrolytes are that bad. Everyone says, "You're gonna die, you're gonna die," but I don't die, so how can it be that dangerous?

*Therapist*: Yeah, that is confusing. [validation] I am sitting here saying there are specific things, like hypokalemia, that have been shown to be life-threatening, *and* you have a history of being told you're going to die but don't. Must be hard to know what to believe.

*Client*: Yeah, I just think we are wasting time on this issue. It hasn't killed me in the past, so. . . .

*Therapist*: I am glad it hasn't killed you in the past. You know, your comment about everyone always telling you you're going to die has me thinking. In my experience, people (like doctors or parents) often use that language broadly and sometimes as a way to scare people into changing. The problem is that many ED symptoms are not imminently life-threatening. They certainly can be very problematic long-term but there are really a very specific set of symptoms that we know can stop your heart or cause acute death. The question is, can you and I agree on what those are and are you willing to stay stable enough—at least for the next four weeks—so you don't die from low potassium.

*Client*: Maybe, I don't know though . . .

*Therapist*: That's okay. Most people need time to decide if this treatment is the best approach for them. In MED-DBT, we rely on international guidelines and published standards to know what is acutely dangerous. I certainly don't want to lump all ED symptoms into that category. Without a doubt, though, hypokalemia is life-threatening. Do you know why?

*Client*: (*Shrugs.*) I don't really know.

*Therapist*: Potassium helps carry electrical signals to the cells in your body. When it's too low, like yours is right now, it means that your nerves and muscles, in particular your heart, are not getting the proper electrical stimulation they need to function.

*Client*: So what are you asking me to do?

*Therapist*: If we decide to work together, I would expect us to work on resolving that instability right away and consult your medical providers to figure that out.

*Client*: Do I need to do all this bloodwork?

*Therapist*: That's the only way I know of to see what your electrolytes are doing. Do you know of another way?

*Client*: Not really.

*Therapist*: So, if we work together, one thing would be getting labs done as needed. In this case, it might mean weekly labs until we see 2–3 consecutive weeks of stable levels of potassium. The bigger picture is agreeing to target medical instability as a primary treatment goal. Of course, there are pros and cons to this. We really need to think this through.

*Client*: I guess. . .

*Therapist*: I do not want to pressure you at all! If you don't agree with doing the tests or the test results or you don't want to resolve medical instability, I don't hold judgment. Do I want to work with you? Yes! And you need to make the choice that is best for you.

*Client*: And if I say no?

*Therapist*: Again, no judgment. It would mean, however, that we can't work together since MED-DBT requires a willingness to work on staying alive. But I can refer you to other types of ED treatment.

*Client*: No, I don't want to see another ED person. So, what do I do? Because I am not ready to stop purging, and I am not sure I want to work on my eating disorder.

*Therapist*: I really appreciate how open and honest you are about what feels safe for you right now. [reinforcement] I am not asking you to commit to full recovery. We haven't even talked about what that would look like or even mean for you. What I am asking for is a willingness on your part to stay stable enough so that you don't die from the ED or any other immediately life-threatening behaviors. I mean, would you be willing to try that over the rest of this pretreatment phase? We haven't even decided whether MED-DBT is the right choice!

*Client*: That actually feels okay, but how do I stay out of risk?

*Therapist*: What would your doctor say you need to do to resolve the hypokalemia?

*Client*: Probably to decrease purging or take supplements.

*Therapist*: Would you be willing to do one or both of those things in an effort to stay alive?

*Client*: I am willing to take potassium supplements, and I can try to reduce purging more.

*Therapist*: I really respect that effort. I know it isn't easy. How can you get the supplements?

*Client*: I need to call my doctor's office.

*Therapist*: Okay, do you want to do that today?

*Client*: Yeah, I will do that.

In this dialogue, the therapist weaves in a number of strategies to increase the client's willingness to stay alive. Psychoeducation is provided, and the therapist maintains a nonjudgmental and collaborative stance even when the client is ambivalent about stopping purging or getting lab work done. Dialectically, the therapist holds that there is validity in both the client's desire not to get labs done *and* in the need to monitor medical stability.

## If Your Client Is Getting Worse during the Pretreatment Phase

Clients in pretreatment are often quite unwell. They have been discharged from day treatment programs and referred from other outpatient therapists due to the severity of their symptoms and an overall lack of success with traditional ED services. Given that you are not their therapist yet and they are not in MED-DBT at this stage, how do you manage risk and declining health over the month while they are in pretreatment? We discussed earlier that rushing clients into MED-DBT is not advised. Providing "some" MED-DBT during pretreatment is also not advised. Instead, therapists remain dialectical, seeking to explore and offer solutions while simultaneously not acting as the individual therapist or case manager. We recommend the following:

1. Validate your client's distress and the discomfort of having to wait four weeks to fully access MED-DBT.
2. Help your client brainstorm ways they can mitigate risk (use of harm reduction strategies) during this phase of treatment (e.g., taking potassium supplements if hypokalemic, reducing activity, or adding in a supplement to help with bradycardia).
3. Discuss a crisis plan for what your client can do should they need additional medical and psychological support during this phase. This might include more frequent medical visits, using crisis lines, accessing nonprofit ED or other services, talking with family about how they can be supportive at this time, or going to the emergency room.
4. Reinforce and shape your client's efforts to address medical instability.
5. Problem-solve how you and the client can effectively manage anxious or angry family members or healthcare providers who may not understand the nature of the pretreatment phase.

## If Your Client Is Medically Unstable and Won't Resolve Instability

There will be times when your client is unable or unwilling to resolve medical instability. When this happens, we use DBT commitment and dialectical strategies to explore ambivalence and enhance commitment without judgment or pressure for clients to agree with us. You can want them to resolve the instability *and* you can't force them into MED-DBT. At these times, it is important not to label your client as resistant or difficult, but rather to see the validity of their experience and to respect their choices. This can be really hard for traditionally trained ED providers (or for those less familiar with EDs in general) who may feel the need to hang on to the client because of the instability regardless of an agreement to resolve that instability.

Your job is to stay dialectical, which means pushing for change and accepting the impasse. It also means observing limits and not extending the pretreatment phase to continue to have repeated discussions about whether or not to target life-threatening ED symptoms. We say this because it can be tempting to remain in this back-and-forth space for months with a client. Not only is this often unhelpful, but it may reinforce the belief that getting support while actively staying unstable is acceptable. Our clients have the freedom to choose whether or not this treatment model is a good fit for them. This means that you have to be willing to let them go when there is an unwillingness to resolve medical stability. This can be an exceptionally difficult situation given that there are few, if any, other viable or preferred treatment options. They may see you as their last hope, which is why it is so important to maintain the stance that treatment cannot work if they are dead. In fact, you believe that to be true to such a degree that you are willing to not proceed without that agreement.

Finally, if your client is unable to achieve medical stability, it may be that they need an environmental intervention such as hospitalization. In these rare cases, it might be recommended that the client receive medical care and then get on the waiting list again for outpatient MED-DBT treatment. In such circumstances, we are allowing the natural contingencies to exist (e.g., they may be unable to stay alive and the only options may be a higher level of care). In our experience, it is the therapist's ability to allow that tension to exist, without resolving it, that shapes clients to choose MED-DBT.

## Identifying Life Worth Living Goals

It would be naive to expect a client to choose life (even temporarily) without a vision of or dream for a different existence. If nothing hangs in the balance, engaging in another treatment might just seem exhausting and futile. All DBT treatments are rooted in the notion of building a "life worth living" which you assess and explore during pretreatment. You may find that some of your clients don't even know how to dream about this, the concept is so foreign or was never made available to them. In Swenson's (2016, p. 7) writing on starting to discuss a life worth living, he states that "initiating the conversation provides a window into the patient's capacity to envision a positive future and work toward it." What, if anything, does your client long for in terms of their future? What would they be doing if they were not dealing with the physical and psychological difficulties they face? Have they come to pretreatment on their own accord or to satisfy someone else's need? This conversation, which begins in pretreatment but extends throughout MED-DBT, is highly nuanced. The concept of building a life worth living takes on new meaning for our clients, most of whom struggle to find acceptance in a dominant culture that praises weight loss and upholds fat-phobic (and other oppressive) attitudes and beliefs. We discuss this in detail in Chapter 10.

## Summary

The MED-DBT pretreatment phase is a highly intentional and structured process designed to increase commitment, enhance client-therapist alignment, and set the foundation for successful engagement in comprehensive treatment. Across four sessions, clinicians work with clients to explore treatment fit, clarify life-threatening risks, and assess whether there is a willingness to stay alive and engage in treatment. Unique to this model is a refusal to rush the process, even in the face of urgency, emphasizing that informed commitment and mutual agreement are essential for long-term success. Clients are not assumed to be "in" treatment until the pretreatment phase is complete, which distinguishes MED-DBT from other ED approaches. This approach honors both the client's agency and the therapist's limits while centering commitment to medical stability, a collaborative alliance, and the possibility of change.

Having established the structure and goals of the pretreatment phase, the next step is to collaboratively develop a shared understanding of the client's difficulties. Chapter 9 outlines how to use the adapted biosocial theory as a compassionate framework for conceptualizing why your client struggles and how symptoms have been reinforced. This chapter provides tools to co-construct that formulation with your client as a central task of pretreatment.

# 9

# Strengthening Commitment
## Later Tasks in MED-DBT Pretreatment

This chapter continues the pretreatment process, with a focus on helping clients make sense of their symptoms through the adapted biosocial theory and determining whether MED-DBT is a good fit. Here, you'll focus on how to introduce the theory in a collaborative and validating way, using the figures and frameworks outlined in Chapters 3 and 4 to co-construct an understanding of why your client struggles and why other treatments may have fallen short. In addition to teaching the theory, this chapter outlines how to orient clients to the key treatment modes of MED-DBT and continue attending to any emerging ambivalence or behavioral patterns that may interfere with engagement. The final task of pretreatment, discussed here, is making a shared decision: Is the client ready and willing to move forward with comprehensive MED-DBT? If so, you will collaboratively identify next steps and transition into active treatment. This chapter helps ensure that you and your client begin treatment with shared clarity, purpose, and momentum.

## Developing a Collaborative Conceptualization Using the MED-DBT Biosocial Theory

A core task of pretreatment is to build a shared and compassionate understanding of your client's difficulties, an understanding that is often missing from previous interventions. As we have highlighted in previous chapters, clients entering MED-DBT frequently carry long histories of unsuccessful treatment attempts, misdiagnoses, and invalidating care experiences. Some have been labeled "chronic" or "resistant," while others have been excluded from services altogether. Many believe nothing will work. This has become especially concerning as, at the time of this writing, there is debate in the field regarding terminality and clinical futility for those who have not responded to standard treatment approaches (Asaria, 2023; Crow, 2023; Guarda et al., 2022). Thus, the adapted biosocial theory serves as a foundational component of MED-DBT, one that directly challenges outdated narratives of futility and offers clients a more compassionate, evidence-informed understanding of their struggles.

Typically introduced in the first session, we orient our clients to the adapted biosocial theory to determine whether, and how, it makes sense to them. The model is a means of restoring hope and making sense of seemingly paradoxical or stuck behavior patterns. Through collaborative conversation, you and your client will explore whether this framework resonates, and if it can offer a new lens on their lived experience. A full description of the MED-DBT biosocial theory can be found in Chapters 3 and 4, and we recommend using the figures provided there as visual aids when explaining the model. We have also included a conceptualization handout you can use with your clients (Handout 9.1). Your approach is one of curiosity and non-judgment: We respect that there is knowledge to be shared by both clinician and client during this process. It is important not to impose your conceptualization of your client onto them, but rather to explore the theory and its possible fit with your client's lived experience without attachment to a specific outcome (i.e., that the client must agree with the conceptualization). If the model doesn't fit with your client's view of themselves, that is okay! Remember that the pretreatment phase is designed to make sure the theories and framework that guide MED-DBT fit for you and your client. If they don't, another treatment pathway will need to be discussed.

## Orient to the Modes, Assumptions, and Interventions Used in MED-DBT

Even if your client is suitable for MED-DBT, agrees with the biosocial theory, and seems like a good fit for individual therapy, they are not ready to start treatment! Your client still needs to learn what to expect in terms of how we will work on reaching their life worth living goals. An informed decision about treatment needs to include agreement on (1) treatment goals and (2) how those goals will be achieved. Often clients are admitted to ED treatments quickly, sometimes involuntarily, and without knowing the specific goals of the program and/or how they are expected to meet those goals. They often find out during the course of treatment what is expected of them. In MED-DBT, we want to make sure our clients have all the information about the theories, assumptions, and interventions we use *before* agreeing to begin. While you and your client may agree on *what* you would like to work on in therapy, you may not agree on *how* you will work on them. For example, your client may want to reduce suicidal behavior and medical instability *and* your client may not be willing to attend skills groups or get labs done. It is imperative that your clients agree on the philosophy, approach, and manner in which we will help them meet their goals. Without a shared agreement, the treatment cannot proceed.

We find that once we have interest in and agreement to the MED-DBT biosocial theory and have identified initial life worth living goals, clients are much more interested in learning how the program will address these areas. By now, your client has already learned a little bit about the target hierarchy (i.e., staying alive is top priority) and they will have been exposed to the style of MED-DBT through the therapist's modeling of treatment assumptions and philosophy. To keep things moving forward, we now introduce clients to the modes of treatment (e.g., individual therapy, skills group training, phone coaching, consulting team), treatment assumptions, and key treatment interventions (e.g., more on the target hierarchy, use of MED-DBT diary cards, and using chain/missing link analysis). During pretreatment, we give our clients a sample diary card and chain analysis worksheet to review and use for practice. They are not expected to do these perfectly, rather to gain exposure to the ways we will be working together in MED-DBT. This allows them to "test out" some of the core strategies we will be using and to ask questions about them before formally beginning treatment.

Your job is to work with your client to determine whether MED-DBT philosophy and treatment interventions align with their unique circumstances, needs, and life worth living goals. We provide a worksheet at the end of this chapter to aid in this process. Subsequent chapters provide detailed descriptions of each of these treatment components. Of note, in order to graduate from pretreatment and move into comprehensive MED-DBT, your client needs to agree with these treatment targets and strategies.

## Discussing Potential Obstacles to the Treatment

As pretreatment sessions unfold, the therapist nonjudgmentally observes and describes thoughts, emotions, or actions on the part of the client, the therapist, or in the broader environment that might interfere (or did interfere historically) with treatment engagement. There will be behaviors that arise in the pretreatment phase that, if not addressed, will interfere with treatment delivery later on. For the purposes of pretreatment, however, we highlight how to manage early treatment obstacles to both set the framework for the program and allow clients to decide for themselves if they are willing to work in this way. The following example illustrates how early obstacles may surface in the pretreatment phase and how they can be addressed in a way that supports client autonomy, validates lived experience, and clarifies the expectations of the MED-DBT model.

*Case Study: Glen*

Glen is a 32-year-old cisgender male with atypical anorexia nervosa (AAN) and BPD. He has had more than 20 years of weight cycling, including periods of chronic dietary restraint in which he has lost more than 60 pounds over the course of several months. He was recently medically unstable (e.g., bradycardia). He engages in self-injury several times per month and has angry outbursts in which he throws his phone or another nearby object. He has been discharged early from past ED treatments due to "severe emotion dysregulation," an inability to control his anger, and an "unwillingness" to follow meal plan recommendations. He states that nobody understands him and that treatments expect him to "just gain weight and be okay with it." He has not filled in a diary card as requested in the first two sessions. He states that the diary card makes him overeat and makes everything worse. He uses cannabis daily and does not want to change this behavior. During the pretreatment phase, Glen expresses anger at the therapist for "taking too long" to get him into treatment. When the therapist explains the medical stability criterion, Glen uses judgmental language about the treatment being too rigid and controlling and he does not agree to getting labs or vitals done. The therapist validates that treatment can feel slow at the start and reviews the rationale for the pretreatment phase. Glen doesn't attend for his third appointment and at the fourth session says that if treatment doesn't start right away, he will leave.

Modeling MED-DBT assumptions about clients, you would communicate your belief that Glen is doing the best he can, that he desperately wants to feel better, *and* that we need to try harder to do this differently or we risk the same poor treatment responses that he has experienced in the past. The conversation might sound like this:

*Therapist*: I am glad you are here today. I wanted to let you know that I appreciate your openness with me about your concerns and distress about the process. You bring up some important things, and I would like us to talk about them today. Is that okay with you?

*Glen*: That's fine, but I don't really want to waste much more of my time.

*Therapist*: I don't want that for you either, and in order for this treatment to have a chance of working, we would need to be on the same page about what we are working on and why.

*Glen*: I just want to get started, no more wasting time.

*Therapist*: Before we can do that, though, we have an even bigger problem to try to solve.

*Glen*: What is that?

*Therapist*: You are angry, much of which makes sense to me. You have been misunderstood, your needs minimized by healthcare providers who didn't take your ED seriously, and you have felt that existing ED treatments were unable to help you. I would be angry too. And your anger is getting in the way of you and I building a connection and a treatment plan.

*Glen*: Well, I am just tired of spending time and money only to end up with nothing in the end.

*Therapist*: That is the exact reason that I am taking this pretreatment time with you—to do everything we can to minimize the chances of that happening again. If you want to see if this approach could help you, and I believe it can, you need to help me carve out a nonjudgmental space for us to talk it through.

*Glen*: Why is everyone on my case about my anger?!

*Therapist*: Probably because you're good at it and it causes people to back off or get angry back at you, and if that happens with us, then the treatment can't survive. You can and likely will be angry or frustrated, and if we are going to work together, we need a way for you to communicate those important feelings without so much fire. The anger gets in the way of us working on your eating and body image concerns.

*Glen*: Fine, I can try that, but I still don't believe that tracking my labs and food intake is helpful. It just makes everything way worse.

*Therapist*: I appreciate the willingness to try, Glen. Thank you. Before we talk about labs and food tracking, can I make another request?

*Glen*: You ask for a lot . . .

*Therapist*: You aren't the first person to say that to me! Okay, next request. I need you at every session. On time. Ready. There is a lot for us to talk about, and this treatment won't work if you aren't here to absorb it.

*Glen*: When I think people don't get me, I don't see the point in showing up much of the time.

*Therapist*: That's a really good thing for me to know about you. So, if you felt that I didn't understand you, the likelihood is high that you won't want to return to session.

*Glen*: Probably.

*Therapist*: Okay, glad I am asking this because I am very human and can guarantee there will be times when I misunderstand you, especially when anger is the main emotion expressed. [fallibility agreement] So here's the ask: Are you willing to show up at every session, including when you feel unheard, and put that on our agenda so we can talk about it? Otherwise, we are going to land in the same place as previous treatment attempts where we never figure this out and you disappear.

*Glen*: I can try.

*Therapist*: That would be great. How does our session feel so far today? Do you feel like I am getting it and hearing you?

*Glen*: Yeah, so far . . .

*Therapist*: Okay, good to know. I am going to continue then if that is alright. I'd like to shift a little here because I am feeling a bit confused about something else. On one hand, you've said that you want to do the MED-DBT program, that's why you came to this clinic, right?

*Glen*: (*Nods head in agreement.*)

*Therapist*: At the same time, you feel strongly that the diary cards and medical monitoring are unhelpful.

*Glen*: Yes. I have tracked my food so many times in my life, and it just makes me hyper-focus on every last thing I eat. I also hate going to my doctor because he always tells me to lose more weight.

*Therapist*: I am so sorry you've had those experiences with your doctor. I can appreciate why you wouldn't want to talk with them. [validation]

*Glen*: If I lose weight, everyone is happy, but then I get sick and treatments expect me to gain weight and eat food and just deal with it.

*Therapist*: That feels like an impossible way to live. [validation]

*Glen*: It is!

*Therapist*: Given what you've experienced, I imagine that my request to monitor food intake and work with your doctor is quite distressing.

*Glen*: I'm just tired of the same stuff over and over again.

*Therapist*: Yeah, I would be too, and it is really hard because treating an eating disorder and addressing eating, weight, and shape is tough. Could we try to talk more about your concerns and feelings about the diary cards and the lab work and see if we can find a way to move forward, a middle ground maybe?

*Glen*: (*Sighs*.) I am okay with that for now.

For our clients, emotional and interpersonal dysregulation (from a biological standpoint) gets in the way of engaging effectively with treatment. It is also true that histories of traumatic invalidation have played a significant role in how they have learned to cope with oppressive and marginalizing environments. Standard ED approaches do not address the profound dysregulation, impact of chronic invalidation, and emotional turmoil our clients experience, all of which are elevated in the ED treatment context. In MED-DBT, the therapist mindfully and nonjudgmentally identifies and addresses the things that get in the way and assesses whether or not there is willingness or ability on the client's part to work on them as treatment goals.

In the dialogue with Glen, the therapist validates what makes sense (e.g., past experiences with healthcare providers around weight and eating have been invalidating and upsetting, and have created mistrust in working with them), normalizes emotions (e.g., anger is functional and is telling you something doesn't feel safe), and nonjudgmentally identifies that getting angry and not doing labs or diary cards will interfere if they were to move forward. The therapist highlights the paradox that Glen is curious about MED-DBT and is saying he can't participate in aspects of it. Glen's emotions and needs are also respected in that the therapist does not impose views or treatment needs on him, rather, creates space to enter into more discussion. Note that the therapist maintains a calm demeanor and does not view Glen's responses as resistant or unwilling, rather maintains the MED-DBT assumptions that he is doing his best given biology and learning history and that he needs to try harder to get a different result.

## Making a Decision and Completing Paperwork

We recognize that making a decision about whether to proceed with treatment is often difficult for the client, the team, or both. By Session four, the client has helped to create a collaborative formulation, understands what the MED-DBT program is and how it links to their unique struggles, and has been presented with a possible path forward. The experience should leave the client feeling validated, affirmed, and valued and, at the very least, with a comprehensive framework for making sense of themselves and the system in which they have been trying to navigate. This is valuable as an intervention in its own right. Now it is time to make a decision about whether or not to move forward.

At the conclusion of this last pretreatment session, if a decision has not been made, the therapist asks the client to think about what they would like to do and gives a specified time frame for when a final decision needs to be made. There is no judgment with respect to ambivalence or the time needed, and MED-DBT therapists observe their own (or their program's) limits with respect to how much time is reasonable to decide. Most programs will give a one- to two-week window. If the therapist needs more help from the team to problem-solve, this is brought to the weekly consult team meeting, and the client is aware of when the therapist will get back to them.

As stated previously, the client is free to choose not to do MED-DBT. It is also true that MED-DBT will not be the right approach for every client. If a client decides against pursuing the treatment, the therapist responds with understanding and genuineness and validates what makes sense about the client's wish not to proceed. The therapist can observe their own desire for the client to stay on without imposing it on the client (e.g., "I have to tell you that I wish you would do this treatment, and I appreciate your position that this doesn't feel like it makes sense for you right now"). The therapist thanks the client for engaging in the pretreatment process, which is an important piece of work on its own, and lets the client know they can reapply to the program at another time should they feel the program might be helpful in the future. We do not want to bring clients into yet another treatment experience that might be invalidating and/or cannot meet their needs.

For us, there are few circumstances that would prevent a client from entering MED-DBT. As detailed above, we would not move forward if the client was not able or willing to resolve medical instability (e.g., not willing to get labs done regularly, not willing to take potassium supplements to protect against hypokalemia). To move forward in the absence of this agreement would likely result in problems, impasses, and increased burnout for both client and therapist as treatment evolves.

We also would like to acknowledge again the emotional load on providers when clients are not responding to the pretreatment work. The desire to "get them into treatment" is pronounced and is one of the reasons why MED-DBT clinicians need support. During these times, we are reminded that standard approaches have not been effective for this patient group. An adherent pretreatment phase is a powerful intervention that builds commitment and engagement to the treatment plan, and in order for it to work, therapists must be willing to let the client go when it isn't a good fit. Clinging to a client who doesn't agree with the philosophy or the modes of therapy is not effective even if there may not be many options for the client. Therapists must practice accepting the difficult reality of the situation with their client and observe the "freedom to choose in the absence of alternatives."

If the client decides to move forward, the therapist reinforces the decision to pursue MED-DBT with warmth and energy while validating that this is still a big commitment. Next steps involve:

1. Reviewing and signing MED-DBT treatment contract documents
2. Confirming with the team that your client will be starting
3. Confirming weekly therapy times
4. Providing information on the time and location of the skills group
5. Providing your contact information for phone coaching

## Summary

Developing a shared conceptualization using the adapted MED-DBT biosocial theory is one of the most validating and clinically powerful parts of the pretreatment phase. For many clients, this is the first time their symptoms have been explained in a way that feels accurate, respectful, and grounded in both science and lived experience. Rather than focusing solely on eating disorder behaviors, this chapter helps clinicians guide clients in exploring the emotional, biological, and environmental factors that have contributed to their suffering. Done collaboratively, this conversation plants the seeds for renewed motivation and hope.

With a shared understanding of the client's struggles in place, the next step is to help them imagine what life could look like beyond those struggles. Chapter 10 focuses on building a life worth living, a central pillar of MED-DBT that allows the therapist and client to align treatment goals with the client's values, desires, and sense of purpose. This process helps create the motivation necessary to move forward into treatment, even when the path ahead feels uncertain or overwhelming.

**Handout 9.1**

## MED-DBT CONCEPTUALIZATION HANDOUT

**Client Name:** ____________________ **Clinician:** ____________________
**Date:** ______________________________

**BIOSOCIAL THEORY:**

| ***Genetic/Neurobiological Factors*** | |
|---|---|
| *Undercontrolled emotion (emotional sensitivity, intensity, slow return to baseline, high reward sensitivity, impulsive, global-processor, BPD diagnosis)* | |
| *Overcontrolled emotion (flat affect, low reward sensitivity, aloof/distant style, inhibited, shy, detail focused, socially isolated, OCPD or ASD diagnosis)* | |
| *Family history of ED* | |
| *Family history of other mental or physical health conditions* | |
| *Sensory or perceptual differences, neurodivergent (e.g., texture, sound, light, touch, taste)* | |
| *Metabolic findings, GI system problems* | |
| *Other:* | |

Copyright © 2026 Anita Federici and Lucene Wisniewski. From *Treating Eating Disorders with DBT* by Anita Federici and Lucene Wisniewski, published by The Guilford Press (2026). Permission to photocopy this material, or to download and print enlarged versions (*www.guilford.com/federici-forms*) is granted to purchasers of this book for personal use or use with others; see copyright page for details.

| *Invalidating Environments* | |
|---|---|
| *Invalidation of emotion and self-regulation qualities* | |
| *Diet culture/weight stigma* | |
| *Denial of problem by caring others* | |
| *Medical minimization/denial* | |
| *Trauma (includes PTSD, sexual, physical, and psychological abuse)* | |
| *White, cisgendered narrative* | |
| *Other:* | |

Life Worth Living Goals :

1. ____________________
2. ____________________
3. ____________________
4. ____________________

| TARGET HIERARCHY<br>*Identify with the client where their current symptoms fall on the target hierarchy. These targets link to the life worth living goals.* | |
|---|---|
| **T1 Life-Threatening:** | |
| **T2 Treatment-Interfering:** | |
| **T3: Quality-of-Life-Interfering:** | |

## DIALECTICAL DILEMMAS

As the conceptualization evolves, make note (with the client) of any of the following secondary treatment targets (e.g., where they show up).

| | |
|---|---|
| Emotional vulnerability versus self-invalidation | |
| Active passivity versus apparent competence | |
| Unrelenting crisis versus inhibited grieving | |
| Apparent compliance versus active defiance | |
| Rigid, overcontrolled eating versus absence of an eating plan | |
| Expecting independence versus fostering dependence | |
| Normalizing pathological behaviors versus pathologizing normative behaviors | |

Therapist Signature and Date: ______________________________

Client Signature and Date: ______________________________

# 10

# The Life Worth Living Discussion

Sam was a 28-year-old veterinarian when she first came to MED-DBT. She had been diagnosed with AN-B/P, BPD, PTSD, and a substance use disorder. She had been in and out of psychiatric care since the age of 17, spanning outpatient, day treatment, and residential treatment. She was in a long-term relationship that was "falling apart" which was causing her a great deal of pain. However, when asked what brought her to the program, she shrugged her shoulders and expressed significant doubt: "I don't really believe anything can help at this point and even if it could, I am not at all sure I want more help. My partner says if I don't get help he will leave me." The therapist validated her long journey, how exhausted and disappointed she might feel at the prospect of "nothing working," and asked more about not wanting more help. She expressed irritation at this question and said, "I am so sick of everyone just expecting me to keep going. Why would I at this point?!" Sam described that past periods of ED recovery were marked by depression, severe body image disturbance, dissociation, and gastrointestinal upset: "If your idea of a life worth living means I have to feel like that, I am not interested."

The ultimate goal in MED-DBT is to help clients build lives that they experience as worth living. The "worth living" part refers to a life that is experienced by your client as satisfying, meaningful, deeply connected to one's values, and brings happiness. Most of what has been written regarding the life worth living (LWL) philosophy has addressed the treatment of chronic suicidal and self-injurious behavior. But what does that mean for someone like Sam who has experienced weight and nutritional stability as the *opposite* of satisfying and happy? What does it mean to pursue an LWL in the context of sociocultural environments that are weight-biased and fat-phobic? How does one feel happy when ED recovery can mean living in a body that feels unfamiliar, unsafe, or is rejected by society, or when eating exacerbates underlying neurobiological disturbances that lead to difficult physical sensations and pain? How does one build an LWL if the family places great value on fitness or clean eating and disagrees with a nondieting philosophy? For these reasons, clinicians working with our clients often tell us that they are unsure how to elicit the LWL discussion in an ED context. This chapter explores ways to describe, define, and discuss an LWL for those with long-standing and multidiagnostic EDs.

## Discussing an LWL with Your Clients

For those coming from a DBT lens, your familiarity and comfort talking about an LWL is a well-established skill set, but we find that the ED often needs more focus in terms of targeting what gets in the way of an LWL for our clients. Therefore, your job will be to broaden your scope to integrate ED knowledge and nuance into the LWL discussion. That means talking with your clients about (and working to resolve) the unique neurobiological and sociocultural challenges they face when attempting to build satisfying and deeply meaningful lives.

For those trained in standard ED approaches, the LWL discussion will feel different and maybe even uncomfortable for two main reasons:

1. *LWL is the treatment priority:* While attention to quality of life is not new to the ED field, it is not the primary driver of traditional ED treatments. CBT, FBT, or hospital-based programs prioritize eating and physical health and view quality of life as a secondary target that will evolve with recovery. Standard treatments make the assumption that an LWL must include full ED recovery (or will come after full recovery). In MED-DBT, building an LWL is the driver of the entire model; it is the vision that drives the treatment, the light at the end of the tunnel, the north star, and the treatment is the blueprint for how to find it. It is the reason for putting oneself through treatment in the first place. Therefore, your job is to help your client develop the LWL "dream" and then use MED-DBT to get them there. ED behaviors are addressed through the lens of the target hierarchy and based on the degree to which they impact LWL.

2. *LWL goes beyond traditional views of ED recovery:* In MED-DBT, we do not define, impose, or make assumptions about what an LWL means or looks like for a client. While we strategically target (and never lose sight of) weight, eating, and ED symptoms, we do not ascribe to narrow definitions of recovery. This may make some of you anxious or uncomfortable. We have to remind ourselves that these are clients for whom standard approaches have not worked. They have already tried (usually multiple times) to engage with treatments that emphasize weight and abstinence as primary goals. In our experience, a dialectical view of our client's goals has been a very meaningful approach for our clients who have felt lost and without direction with more binary views (e.g., recovered versus relapsed). LWL may or may not include full ED recovery at this time. Alternatively, we help our clients pursue the factors, qualities, and conditions they want and need (e.g., achieving independence, having satisfying relationships, feeling safe) in order to experience their lives as rewarding, grounded, and significant.

## Clinician Assumptions That Interfere with the LWL Frame

One assumption is that you can't have this conversation because clients are too ill. While cognitive capacity may be impacted by the ED, your clients are usually very capable of having LWL conversations. In fact, most find it refreshing and welcome the collaborative nature of brainstorming the bigger picture. Another assumption is that focusing on LWL means we are not taking eating and health seriously; occasionally, when starting MED-DBT, providers or family members express concern that we are minimizing the severity of the ED, reinforcing it by not being more aggressive about targeting weight/eating, or that we are downplaying the data on how dangerous the impact to the brain and body of prolonged ED symptoms. Nothing could be further from the truth: MED-DBT was designed specifically with these concerns and issues in mind. We believe that a dialectical treatment focusing on biotemperament is precisely what helps our clients move away from the ED. That said, MED-DBT does require you and your client's family to tolerate a slower rate of change than what you would have expected from standard ED treatments.

The assumption that you do not need to target the ED directly to achieve an LWL is also harmful. Based on our clinical experiences and the research literature to date, we have not been successful in treating both the ED and the emotion regulation difficulties our clients experience in models that do not address the ED: if this were possible, standard DBT would have been sufficient. Our clients need us to be able to understand, appropriately target, and help them manage an ED in the context of suicide, self-injury, and pervasive emotional instability.

## Eliciting the Dream

We all search for meaning, crave a sense of purpose, and feel more grounded when we are living according to our values. So how do we help our clients build, define, and dream about *their* LWL without imposing our own biases, beliefs, or expectations on them? The LWL is the *why*. For example, if a client's LWL goal includes having a fulfilling job and relationship, do they need to change their ED behaviors in order to have these? It is generally not enough to say, "I want to purge less." The *why* is what helps to carry our clients through when things get tough: "I want to purge less because when I purge a lot I get unstable and then I have to go to a higher level of care and then will lose the job/relationship that I like." This is in contrast to the approach of "We must address all ED symptoms because you have an ED."

Some clients will come with ideas and desires. Others will have never entertained the idea of an LWL or will not want to entertain discussions about hope and dreams after many experiences of being let down. Moreover, for our clients, the LWL discussion is tricky because the ED often feels like the only viable LWL path. Clients have reported feeling an increase in suffering when they are weight restored or that their urges for suicide increase with the elimination of ED behaviors: "I felt so much worse after I gained weight because all the emotional pain I didn't have to feel when starving came back, and worse. More dysregulated, more intense for being squashed down so long, and more frightening. All the security I gained from restriction, gone" (Downs, 2021, p. 3).

Talking about an LWL cannot be a superficial or one-off conversation. It requires you to deeply understand the way our clients have felt lied to or otherwise deceived by the promise of standard treatment approaches. This is also similar to a related kind of invalidation, as the people around your client may have expressed relief thinking that their loved one is "better" now that they have stopped engaging in behaviors. In our case example at the beginning of the chapter, Sam can't imagine a satisfying or safe life without the ED *and* this doesn't mean you can't help her try to find one. As described by Swenson (2016, p. 7), "Initiating the conversation provides a window into the patient's capacity to envision a positive future and work toward it."

## Cultivating Motivation

MED-DBT providers maintain a paradoxical approach to cultivating motivation: (1) we need our clients to pursue the goal of staying alive and to build a LWL, (2) we accept that our clients may not want to choose life or build an LWL, and (3) we do not drag a client through treatment. Let's break this down.

On one hand, we uphold a tenacious position and always choose life as a necessary precursor to building an LWL. A shared agreement that one needs to be alive in order to achieve a meaningful life is like accepting that building a new house requires a strong foundation from which the rest of the house is constructed. A house without a foundation has a great likelihood of sinking, breaking apart, and crumbling to the ground. So, we need the basic building blocks (e.g., the LWL dream) to exist if we want to build and sustain a quality life for our clients. At the same time, we radically accept that wanting to stay alive is usually not what our clients want when we first meet them. Our clients have suffered with little reprieve for many years, and our ask to choose life at all costs can seem invalidating—why would we ask them this if we understood how painful their lives have been? For many clients, efforts to eliminate the ED and stabilize weight have resulted in body sensations that feel intolerable, sociocultural repercussions, and/or intense emotional suffering and suicidality. However, life with ED is equally painful (though perhaps more predictable). Our clients have not been able to find a middle ground, and instead have moved from one type of distress to another. Lost between an untenable set of symptoms and an as yet unachieved LWL, we acknowledge that the thought of death may have been experienced as a reprieve, an escape, and a solution.

The unwavering position to choose life is held, dialectically, with the position that we do not drag clients into or through MED-DBT. In spite of our desire to hang on to a client, we cannot proceed with treatment if our client is not willing or able to be a part of the process. This can be a source of tension in our field as some argue that ED treatment cannot wait for collaboration, particularly in light of presentations marked by a starved brain and/or lack of insight into the severity of the illness that so many of our clients experience. The application of this assumption does not mean that a client has to be in a place to agree with every aspect of recovery. It means that we seek to identify a common ground and to and to *nurture commitment through collaboration* in the work of staying alive. Take, for example, a 22-year-old client who tells you they do not want to work on eating, weight stability, or self-injury but wants their parents to leave them alone so they can return to university. An expression of this assumption might sound like the following:

"I could be very helpful to you in getting your parents off your back and getting you to school ***and*** I wouldn't be able to achieve that without you joining me in the process. I am also guessing that the medical instability and the repeated hospitalizations reinforce your parent's behavior to never let go. If we work on staying alive, that could very well solve these two problems and it is, of course, your choice to move forward in that way."

Our clients are typically not accustomed to this style of engagement. The very nature of a multidiagnostic ED presentation draws fear, panic, and frustration from families, peers, clinicians, and hospital programs. Our clients are usually told what to do, have been involuntarily admitted at times, and/or have felt that treatment is something "done to them," rather than "with them." Ironically, the MED-DBT stance is often experienced as empowering and highly validating to clients, and it sets the stage for a co-created path forward. Thus, big picture life goals emerge for your client while you dialectically explore the middle ground between suicide/wanting to die from the ED versus building a LWL without dragging them to see it your way. As the therapist, you

> have to be able to "get into hell" with the patient and see what it looks and feels like, and to help the patient "find a way out of hell." . . . It's a synthesis of acceptance and change. The work of "finding a way out of hell" begins with the work of envisioning a life worth living that works for that patient. (Swenson, 2016, p. 13)

There isn't one way to get at the LWL dream; how you elicit it depends on your client and your conceptualization. We have provided some ideas here to get you started.

- "If you were to allow yourself to dream even a little bit, how would your life be different? What would you want? If the ED wasn't holding you back, what would your life look like?"

- "Did you have ideas or dreams when you were young about what you wanted your life to be/look like?"
- "What is important for me to know about/for us to consider in terms of your gender or cultural background when we think about an LWL?"
- "How does diet culture influence your idea of an LWL?"
- "Have you ever experienced your life as deeply meaningful and satisfying? When was that? What factors made it feel that way?"
- "Whom do you admire? Why? What is it about the way they live that you feel drawn to?"
- "Do you have specific life values or spiritual beliefs that are important to you?"
- "How do you know if you are not living according to your values?"
- "If you felt really well, stable, and grounded, what would you be doing? Who would be in your life? Where would you live?"
- "If a good friend were hosting your 80th birthday party, what would you want them to focus on about you and your life in their celebratory speech?"
- "Beyond the ED, what has interfered with pursuing or maintaining an LWL?"

Notice that some of these utilize a door-in-the-face strategy while others operate from a foot-in-the-door approach. As you have these conversations with your client, you develop a more nuanced understanding of how their behaviors and environment have helped and hindered their dreams. Remember not to fall into the either–or trap—for example, "Well, you can't really have those things if you aren't fully recovered." It is more nuanced than that—for example, "I love hearing you talk about your vision of moving to the coast and finding a way to help others. I would be really interested to hear more about what helps you get closer versus farther away from that dream."

## Commitment Strategies

In this section, we highlight how we use commitment strategies over the course of MED-DBT to stay focused on building lives worth living. While the LWL discussion defines the pretreatment phase, it permeates the entire treatment and when the going inevitably gets tough, you will need to connect and reconnect to your client's LWL vision to keep moving forward. It is the big *why* for everything the client is doing in this treatment.

## Pros and Cons

Many clients have come to anticipate suicide, self-injury, ED symptoms, and repeated hospitalizations as a way of life. While this may seem chaotic and turbulent, many with multidiagnostic ED presentations are hesitant to let the ED go: It becomes an identity, a familiar friend, a source of mastery, and a way to soothe an unsettled biology. Much has been written about the strong sense of loyalty to the ED and more broadly pervasive ambivalence about change. The ED can serve as an escape from the demands of life or can be a way to avoid hoping for an LWL (e.g., "I need to be in treatment so I can't do *x*, *y*, or *z*"). As discussed, the ED serves many functions both in terms of biology—such as regulating a disrupted metabolism, coping with complex sensory and perceptual differences, or moderating an emotionally sensitive system—and environment (e.g., regulating the impact of diet culture and weight bias, creating interpersonal boundaries and communications, and coping with other invalidating systems). Thus, in order to talk about an LWL, you must first understand and appreciate the benefits of *not* changing.

It is extremely important to genuinely appreciate the pros and cons of your client's behaviors, especially the ones you don't like. While many therapists report using pros and cons as a motivational strategy, it is often the case that the therapist's bias for which side of the argument they believe the client should choose is quite clear. For example, you might talk with Sam about the pros and cons of starting yet another treatment despite many unsuccessful attempts. You validate the function (the pros) of staying the same but at the end of the session, hope and expect for her to choose to work with you/do it or see it your way. The pros and cons strategy in DBT is not to decide what the "right" answer is, *rather* to elucidate both sides of the change coin without the expectation of resolving it or for your client to see it your way. We usually start with the pros of *not* getting better, with the goal of genuinely understanding just how hard it would be for this person to work on change at this time. It is important to communicate to your client that you are genuinely willing and able to hear all sides, and to recognize the validity in maintaining the status quo.

Let's say Sam is ambivalent during pretreatment about working on medical stability and the session is coming to an end. You would tolerate the urge to force a commitment and instead respect her autonomy and her choice to think about it or to choose not to work on medical stability. An example of what you might say could be:

"Sam, I appreciate your perspective that focusing on staying alive is a significant commitment [*cons of changing*] and maybe not something you want to do right now [*pros of staying the same*]. As I've gotten to know you, I can see how the ED and getting admitted to the hospital give you a much needed break from the stress going on at home with your partner [*pros of staying the same*]. What a tough place to be in (*cons of not changing*). Why don't you take one more week to think about what you want to do and I will see you on Thursday to finish up pretreatment. We'll decide then if MED-DBT makes sense to pursue [*cons of not changing means this treatment will end*]."

## Playing Devil's Advocate

DBT therapists are known for their irreverent and unorthodox ways of responding. A central strategy within DBT is to engage in ways that your client is not expecting in an effort to keep them slightly off balance. Playing devil's advocate means that you purposely take an opposing or contentious position that can have the effect of testing the strength of your client's stance. Remember that a big focus in MED-DBT is on the moment-by-moment transactions between you and your client. When Sam says she doesn't care if she dies, doesn't want to be in ED treatment, and just wants to get back to her busy veterinarian job where she can "lose all the weight she wants," she is likely to be on the receiving end of two dominant responses: (1) an increase in caring and warmth from others combined with a strong pull to convince her to live or to stay in treatment and/or be involuntarily admitted to hospital; and (2) frustration, exacerbation, judgment, or a withdrawal of warmth from others.

Using a devil's advocate strategy, you could respond to Sam in a manner that is different from typical responses. Without judgment and with genuine curiosity, you might say:

"Oh, shoot, I didn't realize you already made up your mind! Hmmm . . . sounds like you already have a plan that doesn't include me. I kind of see what you are getting at. Why bother to put so much effort into yet another treatment, especially one that requires you to agree to stay alive? That sounds like a ton of effort." When done effectively, the response you (hopefully) get back is usually "but I have to because I can't keep going like this."

## Foot-in-the-Door/Door-in-the-Face

Drawing from techniques that defined door-to-door sales, these two strategies are often used together in the face of ambivalence. "Foot-in-the-door" is a technique in which you make a small request that almost anyone would agree to and then build from there. "Door-in-the-face" is the opposite approach, in which you ask for the moon, expecting a rejection, but then land on a synthesis between the current state and the "big ask." Let's pick up where we left off with Sam.

*Therapist*: Sounds like you are in limbo about what to do. Would you be willing to talk more about what would be involved if you decided to do the program? [foot-in-the-door]

*Sam*: I guess so, but I really think this idea of focusing on the eating disorder is overkill, and it has never worked in the past so I am definitely not up for doing that again.

*Therapist*: I appreciate the honesty. I also think there is a difference between going for full ED recovery versus resolving medical stability so you don't die and working toward a life worth living. [foot-in-the-door]

*Sam*: When you put it that way, it sounds more realistic for me.

*Therapist*: I mean, we could push for stopping all ED behaviors right away. Lots of research out there to support that as the main direction. [door-in-the-face]

*Sam*: Yeah, been there, done that. Like I said, I would be willing to stay alive. I get that part, but I am not willing to commit to treating my whole ED at this time and maybe never.

*Therapist*: That can work for us. Can we talk more about what it means for you to stay alive from an ED lens? [foot-in-the-door]

Moving back and forth between these two techniques helps to avoid polarization and increases willingness to find a collaborative and behaviorally specific set of goals that will support building an LWL.

## Linking to Prior Commitments

Building the LWL dream with your client is the lifeline you will rely on later in treatment when ambivalence dominates and the motivation wanes. Sam has had a decade's worth of treatment, doubts whether anyone or anything can help, is on the verge of losing her partner, and has missed many days of work due to past hospitalizations. She has a trauma history, is emotionally vulnerable, has relied on substances to manage intense feelings, and is terrified to experience the sensory discomfort that comes with weight gain. At one point about 10 weeks into treatment, Sam got into an argument with her partner after a difficult weekend marked by many symptoms. When she attended the next session, she had a new bandage on her arm and disclosed that she hadn't eaten for more than 10 hours. She said she was feeling hopeless.

*Sam*: I am done. You're very nice and all, but this treatment is not working and I am so tired.

*Therapist*: I'm so glad you actually came in today to tell me what happened over the weekend and how you are feeling now.

*Sam*: I really just came to tell you that I don't want to do this treatment anymore.

*Therapist*: What?!

*Sam*: Yeah, well I am too tired to deal with the hard stuff.

*Therapist*: After the weekend you've had, I can only imagine how drained and exhausted you must feel. I am also remembering our talks earlier about working through these times together.

*Sam*: I said that when I was feeling better.

*Therapist*: That is probably true! Do you think that was your wise mind back then saying you wanted to stay in treatment even when it got hard?

*Sam*: Oh, probably. I don't have a wise mind anymore.

*Therapist*: I definitely know that wise mind can seem to disappear when life hands us lemons, and I know one of your LWL goals is to improve your relationship and keep your job and not have to go back to the hospital.

*Sam*: It was . . . it is! But I am so gutted by everything that just happened!

*Therapist*: Of course, yes! And I would hate for you to ignore your wise mind here and lose an opportunity to handle this in a way that keeps you in line with your values and life goals. Can we agree to honor our agreement to stay in this together?

## Freedom to Choose in the Absence of Alternatives

A powerful intervention in its own right, emphasizing the freedom to choose is a very important position to hold in this treatment. Your client gets to choose whether they want to work with you or not, whether they want to stay alive or not, whether they eat, stop purging, gain weight, focus on suicide or not—*and* there are natural consequences to those choices.

For example, let's say Sam was taken to the emergency room after fainting at work and admitted to the hospital due to medical instability. She is discharged and attends therapy with you as scheduled two days later. When you ask her for more information and the hospital notes regarding medical instability, she tells you it isn't necessary as "everything is fine now" and she is not willing to talk more about what happened.

In MED-DBT, we respect Sam's right to choose not to tell us even though that might:

- Destabilize the therapy given that we are talking about an unwillingness to discuss possible T1 behaviors
- Impact the therapeutic relationship as it might push your limits
- Take up session time talking about the pros and cons of not disclosing the information instead of talking about a relationship difficulty she wants to discuss

Freedom to choose in the absence of alternatives may well be the hardest commitment strategy to uphold in MED-DBT. When our clients are physically unwell, malnourished, and at risk of medical instability, often the urge is not to give them freedom to choose. We believe that doing something is always better than doing nothing. We assume that using freedom to choose is equivalent to doing nothing (which is not true!). We are afraid that if we observe a limit, our client might die. We assume that the client cannot make decisions. We get shaped by system and familial pressures to keep trying at all costs. We have difficulty allowing natural consequences to influence and shape our clients over time. Sam can absolutely and without judgment decide not to share her medical report from the ER or tell you why she was hospitalized, *and* you can't proceed to help her build an LWL if you don't know if she is at imminent risk of death. Even though there is validity to her decision (there are always multiple truths), it is unfair for Sam to ask you to go ahead without knowing what happened. This is analogous to having a surgery date scheduled, having a medical crisis arise, and not being willing to share the details with your surgeon, even though it might impact your surgery. For those trained in standard DBT, this would be equivalent to knowing your client made a suicide attempt but they are unwilling to discuss the details or do a BCA (behavior-chain analysis) with you. They can decide to do that and there are natural outcomes of that position (e.g., pushing the therapist's limits, decreasing collaboration in the therapeutic relationship).

At another point in treatment, Sam started to lose weight. While restricting her food and fluid intake itself was not T1 or T2 at the time, it was having a big impact on her partner, who became anxious and frustrated (T3). "I am not in the hospital," she would say. "I don't know why he can't just let me live." The therapist, using freedom to choose, responded by saying, "It sounds like not changing your intake will have an impact on your relationship." Staying mindful of your own urge to tell the client that she *needs* to stop losing weight or that the ED is taking over, you help her observe the choices she is making and the subsequent consequences. Similar to pros and cons, you often do not need to resolve the dilemma for your client, instead allowing the tension between two desired outcomes (wanting to lose weight and wanting harmony in her relationship) to create the synthesis for moving forward ("I'd better not lose more weight right now because it impacts him whether I want it to or not, and I don't want that for us").

## Summary

Defining and envisioning an LWL is paramount to the success of MED-DBT: Building and sustaining an LWL is the primary goal that drives the entire treatment. For our clients, the LWL picture must take into account the unique neurobiological and sociocultural factors that shape and influence their lives. It is essential to consider how to build an LWL in a weight-obsessed culture and/or within a body that can feel foreign or unsafe without the ED. These factors cannot be downplayed, as they will unavoidably show up and threaten to stand in the way of progress if not adequately addressed. Therapists are cautioned against perpetuating beliefs that "everything will get better if you just eat/gain weight/stop purging." DBT commitment strategies help us navigate these nuanced waters more successfully and collaboratively both during the pretreatment phase and throughout the duration of treatment.

Of course, envisioning an LWL is only the beginning. Clients must also take concrete steps toward building it. But when multiple problems compete for attention, it can be difficult to know where to begin. In the next chapter, we introduce the MED-DBT target hierarchy: a structured, collaborative framework that helps therapists and clients organize complexity, prioritize interventions, and stay aligned with the ultimate goal of building a life worth recovering into.

# 11

# What to Target and When

Jules (they/them) is a 27-year-old nonbinary individual who presented with atypical anorexia, long-standing suicidal and self-injurious behavior, PTSD, and substance abuse. Jules currently skips breakfast and lunch, walks up to 4 hours per day, and reports binge eating followed by self-induced vomiting at least twice per week. They recently lost 35 pounds. At a recent medical visit, they had a heart rate of 48 beats per minute, orthostatic blood pressure, and their sodium and potassium levels were in the low range of normal. They disclosed to you that they took a potassium supplement prior to the labs because they "didn't want to get admitted to the hospital again."

Jules reports a history of sexual assault and notes that previous attempts at ED treatment didn't adequately address their trauma symptoms. They report that self-injury is typically triggered by PTSD symptoms or GI distress, and/or body hatred. Jules uses cannabis four days a week and occasionally uses alcohol and/or cocaine (once a month). They do not feel that the substance use is problematic; rather, they view it as harm reduction. Jules lives an hour away from your treatment center and is unable to drive due to a license suspension for a DUI.

Jules is seeking treatment for PTSD and is wary about trying MED-DBT because they have "already tried DBT and it didn't work." Jules has a 10-year treatment history that has included FBT, CBT-ED, DBT skills groups, ED day treatment, and various inpatient admissions due to suicide or medical instability. Jules does not consider the ED to be a concern and feels that the lack of focus on PTSD is why they aren't getting better. They report feeling angry with previous ED treatment providers who were not willing to treat trauma and "only focus on the ED." Jules did seek out another provider who attempted to use CPT (cognitive processing therapy); however, said it "blew up" because "the therapist didn't know what to do when I lost a bunch of weight." Of note, Jules tells you that they have felt unsafe and marginalized in most treatment settings, citing a lack of affirming care. They shared the experience of being in an ED program that considered "being nonbinary a part of the eating disorder." Jules is unsure whether MED-DBT will help and whether they can trust you to be a safe and affirming provider.

When faced with multiple problem behaviors and competing needs or expectations, the typical outcome is for client and therapist to get stuck between "Everything is important to target" versus "Only the things *I* think are important should be targeted." The "I" in this statement can be the patient, the family, the therapist, or even the healthcare system. In MED-DBT, the target hierarchy removes the battle over who is right versus wrong with respect to what to focus on and when. Designed to be collaborative in nature, the hierarchy is a shared agreement about how to organize the chaos and move forward with the mutual intention of building an LWL.

If you are coming from a DBT background, the rationale for and use of the target hierarchy is not new. We suspect that the bigger learning curve for you will be in determining where ED behaviors fall on the hierarchy. In many standard DBT programs, we have observed that ED behaviors are either not included in the hierarchy or are added in ways that are not conceptually appropriate (e.g., always putting food restriction as T1 or viewing any purging as T2).

For our colleagues coming from traditional ED approaches, the target hierarchy will be a significant shift in terms of which ED behaviors are targeted and when. Traditional ED treatments would focus on all ED symptoms, with the primary aim of stabilizing weight and nutrition and eliminating compensatory behaviors (e.g., excessive exercise, vomiting, food rituals). As you will see in this chapter, the MED-DBT hierarchy has a much more nuanced and dialectical manner of approaching symptoms that takes into account the ED in the context of the biosocial contributions that influence a given client. This model is based on building a life worth recovering into; thus, targeting is linked to that goal rather than a laser focus on ED behaviors. To date, most of the literature on the DBT hierarchy focuses on the management of suicide and self-injurious behavior. Thus, this chapter provides a detailed description of when and how to target ED symptoms in MED-DBT.

## Target 1: Life-Threatening Behaviors

The lives of our clients are often permeated by suicide, self-injury, and ED-related medical instability. Most have been in and out of treatment settings and emergency rooms, and many will feel that death is the only way to escape from the physical and emotional turmoil that has defined much of their lived experiences. Perhaps one of the most primary dialectical tensions you will hold with your client is the deeply compassionate acceptance of their suffering and desire to end their pain alongside the steadfast belief that they don't want to die. The notion of escaping from pain or disappearing from suffering is not unique to those living with EDs. To dream or fantasize about getting away from stress, grief, and life difficulties is part of the human condition and can serve a robust protective function. At the same time, we also hold the belief that our clients do not want to die, but instead want relief from their suffering. We believe that, given a chance to feel better, they may, in fact, choose life. We view behaviors such as suicidal communication and medical instability as the result of complex situations that have often been reinforced as (temporary) ways of soothing biology (e.g., starvation can calm the GI tract), regulating emotion (e.g., exercising when medically unstable can reduce shame or anxiety), or managing the invalidating environment (e.g., receiving more warmth and caring when hospitalized). The desire to hang onto these coping methods makes sense *and* hanging on also blocks the potential for a different outcome.

The primary aim of MED-DBT is to build an LWL. You cannot help your client do that if they are actively committed to ending their lives. Thus, working together in MED means a collaborative stance in which you and your client agree to target behaviors that could imminently lead to death (T1 behaviors). T1 behaviors in standard DBT include suicidal and self-injurious behaviors. Standard DBT, however, is silent on when ED symptoms become life-threatening. Given the high mortality rates for those with EDs, the MED-DBT hierarchy extends the original Target 1 category to include all ED behaviors when they become acutely life-threatening (and this is not easy for most therapists to determine!).

Navigating the medical landscape of EDs can be confusing for therapists since a myriad of medical complications can range from mild and annoying to severe and life-threatening. Moreover, practitioners using MED-DBT are typically not physicians or nurses so it is not always possible to know when ED behaviors are imminently life-threatening without medical consultation. While certain physical symptoms can be life-threatening (e.g., bradycardia, electrolyte imbalances, heart arrhythmias), medical consultation is needed to fully understand lab results. We also have to keep in mind that science can change as our understanding of what leads to imminent risk evolves. Thus the MED-DBT therapist must (1) be trained to know signs, symptoms, and what can cause acute risk; (2) stay within their scopes of practice; and (3) work with the client to monitor medical stability. In order to accomplish these goals, we use a set of guidelines and steps to determine what constitutes a T1 ED behavior:

1. Evidence of clear (or possible) medical instability via lab work, vitals, symptom reports (e.g., chest pain, fainting). In patients with significant restriction, abdominal pain, nausea, or vomiting may be an indicator of acute gastric dilation as per Anderson, Watters, Dee, and Mehler (2023).
2. Cross-reference the AED Medical Care Guidelines. Published as a brief information package for primary care physicians, the fourth edition of the guidelines was published in 2021 and outlines risk assessment, necessary medical tests, and criteria for acute hospitalization.
3. Refer to other published guidelines. Given the evolving nature of ED risk management, it is important to stay up-to-date with assessment and risk management recommendations in the field. Reviewing newly published articles and attending conference presentations in this area is important.
4. Consultation to the client to determine how to get clear on whether a symptom is acute. For example, your client might call their doctor to clarify the lab work during a session, book an urgent appointment with their physician, go to a medical care clinic, or seek consultation via email from experts in the field.
5. Reflect! Determine if the behavior is T1, T2, or T3. For example, your client has a prolonged QTc interval—a heart rhythm measurement that, when elevated, increases the risk of serious cardiac events such as arrhythmia or sudden cardiac arrest. She works closely with an ED-trained psychiatrist who tells you they are aware of the issue and are medically managing it with your client. You, however, continue to feel very anxious and want your client to get lab work done every week in spite of what her doctor recommends. In this case, you have managed the behavior from a T1 perspective by getting clarity from an ED specialist. The anxiety you are feeling would be better conceptualized

as therapy-interfering, and we would recommend bringing that to your consult team to discuss further.

We appreciate that you might prefer to have a more concrete list of T1 behaviors, *and* criteria for medical stability isn't always clear. It is crucial that you stay dialectical and not overload the T1 category with behaviors that are actually T2 (therapy-interfering) or T3 (quality of life-interfering) behaviors. It is also important to focus on the behavior causing the instability and not the outcome. For instance, bradycardia is not the target, it is the outcome of behavior; you would target the behavior that leads to the instability (e.g., starvation). You might ask your client to increase food and fluid intake or remain on bed rest until they are no longer bradycardic. Thus, restrictive eating may be T1 if it is associated with the presence of bradycardia but not all restricting is T1. Vomiting may be T1 if your client has low potassium, or it may be T2 or T3.

That said, ED symptoms that might not typically be T1 can become imminently life-threatening under certain conditions. For example, exercising is not usually T1, but exercising with a prolonged QTc interval can be. Diet pills (e.g., ephedrine) may become T1 if they cause tachycardia or orthostasis. Therefore, you and your client need to work together to track and resolve these symptoms over the course of treatment with the help of your medical colleagues.

## What to Do If There Is No Doctor or If the Doctor Is Not Responsive to the Labs/Vitals

Given that the average physician has less than 5 hours of ED training, if any, the reality is that most of you will encounter situations in which your client does not have a doctor who accurately understands EDs and minimizes medical risks. In addition to the suggestions on building the MED-DBT team in Chapter 6, the absence of a physician does not mean we ignore T1 behaviors. Your client may need to go to a walk-in clinic, use a virtual medical service, or email experts in the field to get the information needed to determine medical risk. This may also be true should a medical provider dismiss lab results or physical symptoms. For example, a client we worked with started to lose weight, resulting in bradycardia and dizziness. Together with the client, we sent a letter to the treating physician explaining the worsening ED symptoms and the low heart rate detected on the client's watch. The doctor did not respond and when the client called the office to follow up, they were only able to book an appointment five weeks out. The client began binge eating and purging several times per day and started to complain of a sensation of cramping in her chest and upper back. The client went to the emergency room and was admitted for 48 hours for fluids and observation. At discharge, she returned to daily binge/purge behaviors.

Using a consultation-to-the-client approach, we worked together to problem-solve the need for ongoing medical support, and another letter was sent to the doctor's office. The doctor ordered blood tests and the client's potassium was 2.4 but the doctor still did not respond. The lack of response was treatment-interfering, as was the confusion regarding why a low potassium level was being ignored. The heightened anxiety in the treating therapist started to lead to some polarizing conversations with the client, which was therapy-interfering as well. Together with the team, a number of recommendations were made including advocating for the client more strongly given the power dynamics, helping the client access medical services elsewhere, and accessing a case consultation with an outside medical expert.

## How Often Should We Be Collecting Labs/Vitals?

The frequency of lab work depends on the status of your client's health and symptoms, their medical history, and the degree to which lab work links to the target hierarchy. We don't want to arbitrarily collect labs and vitals just because the person has an ED. Some of our guidelines include the following:

1. Recent labs are helpful. You can't know by looking at someone whether they are medically stable, and your client may not feel unwell. When starting out with a new client, getting recent labs that include an ECG gives you a snapshot of their baseline status. If your client recently had lab work done, asking for a copy may be enough.
2. Getting labs and vitals done during the pretreatment phase can alert you and your client to any current concerns, which gives you an opportunity to demonstrate where symptoms would fall on the hierarchy and how they would be addressed if you both move forward with MED-DBT.
3. While behaviors fluctuate in frequency or duration, when ED symptoms change or intensify, you may want new labs/vitals done to ensure your client is stable.

4. Lab work may also be indicated if your client reports physical symptoms (e.g., fainting, abdominal pain, chest pain), starting a new medication (e.g., Seroquel can increase QTc intervals), or having a procedure done (e.g., client undergoing cancer treatment).

T1 behaviors can be hard to detect; therefore, teaching your client how to manage their illness so they are not at risk of dying is an important part of this work. Working collaboratively, you and your client seek clarity on what constitutes medical stability and then target the behaviors the maintain the higher risk. How do Jules's symptoms fit with targeting T1 behaviors? Jules has both bradycardia (heart rate at 48 beats/minute) and orthostatic hypotension. While their electrolytes were reported in the "normal" range, they disclosed taking potassium supplements before the blood test, which would have resulted in a false reading. An updated lab test would be necessary.

Jules also does not want to work on the ED and is very motivated to work on PTSD to reduce suffering. We won't be very effective at getting Jules to trauma treatment if they are dead; therefore, Jules needs to be willing to talk with their doctor about monitoring and resolving medical instability. We are asking them to collaborate on the goal of not dying. The focus is on Jules doing everything in their power to stay alive. While weight gain might be an unintended consequence of resolving medical instability, it is not the goal right now.

## Target 2: Treatment-Interfering Behaviors

Many T2 behaviors in MED-DBT are the same as those observed in standard DBT. As they have been detailed elsewhere (e.g., Linehan, 1993; Heard & Swales, 2015; Chapman & Rosenthal, 2015), we will not extensively cover those here. Instead, this section describes client and clinician ED-specific treatment-interfering behaviors (TIBs) that we commonly encounter in our work.

"Treatment-interfering behaviors" refer to any behavior on the part of the client, family, therapist, or system that interferes with treatment delivery or engagement. Just like in standard DBT, TIBs are the second-highest priority in MED-DBT. Traditional ED approaches do not have the theoretical scaffolding or defined processes for managing the things that "get in the way" of treatment delivery. Yet, as Linehan (1993) wrote, "a therapy applied but not received will fail" (p. 132). Given that outcomes are greatly reduced when clients cannot receive a full course of treatment, we prioritize addressing behaviors that interfere with the treatment.

It is true that our clients and the clinicians who treat them have a much higher likelihood of engaging in behaviors that interfere with treatment engagement and delivery. However, it is not because our clients are "difficult," "treatment resistant," or "unmotivated to change," and it is not because the therapists don't want to treat them! Rather, our clients struggle with emotional and interpersonal dysregulation and/or co-occurring illnesses for which standard approaches were never designed to manage. The clinicians who treat them also report feeling unsure how to manage severe or enduring ED presentations and report more burnout when working with our clients. Thus both clients and therapists need help! Unlike standard ED approaches, we focus on the behaviors that interfere with the dose of treatment, which at times *may* be ED symptoms or could be other behaviors as outlined in this chapter. This means being able to tolerate not working on some ED symptoms when there are other T1 or T2 behaviors present.

Note that it is crucial to approach TIBs with compassion and to demonstrate to your clients your understanding that these behaviors developed as ways to cope (not as ways to "manipulate" or "seek attention"). Even the most challenging or egregious TIBs developed over time have important functions for your clients, and have likely been highly reinforced. When teaching, discussing, or observing TIBs please keep the following in mind:

- *Be nonjudgmental.* It is important not to use the words "therapy-interfering" in a pejorative manner. Teach your client about the origin and intention of the terminology, and model talking about TIBs as a term used to observe and describe behavior. It is essential to see our colleagues and clients through a phenomenological empathic lens.
- *Normalize.* We *all* engage in TIBs, not just our clients. We have observed that most ED outcome studies report on what the client or the caregivers are doing that renders treatments unsuccessful (e.g., the client is suicidal, depressed, aggressive). Treatment is a transaction between two or more people. To focus only on what the client is doing would be non-dialectical. TIBs are commonly observed in clinicians, teams, families, and in organizations. In our treatment, we monitor and target the behavior of the client *and* the therapist that interferes with treatment engagement or delivery.

- *Assess the function.* TIBs are patterns of behavior that have been reinforced, internally or externally, and serve as powerful coping mechanisms. It is important not to make assumptions about these behaviors and to use chain analyses to explore how the behaviors arise and are maintained in yourself and your client.
- *Collaboratively problem-solve.* Do not assume your client or team member knows how to change a TIB. Your job is to be curious and to create a collaborative space to observe, describe, and problem-solve.

## TIBs of MED-DBT Clients

This section expands on T2 client behaviors that can interfere with treatment. Note that we have chosen to maintain Linehan's original TIB categories. In writing this book, we discussed whether to remove certain terms (e.g., "noncollaborative behavior"), as we did not want them to be used in a pejorative or invalidating manner. Our decision to maintain the original descriptors rested on the fact that clinicians have reported that these categories help them to more accurately understand and identify what gets in the way of treatment. In no way do we condone the use of these terms as client descriptors or characteristics. We *all* engage in nonattentive, noncollaborative, and noncompliant behaviors as outlined in this section of the book.

### Category 1: Behaviors That Interfere with Receiving Therapy

"Nonattentive behaviors" refer to thoughts, emotions, and actions that interfere with attending and/or being present during treatment. This includes missing or arriving late to sessions, falling asleep during skills group, threatening to stop therapy, or talking about suicide with people who can legally admit them to the hospital as this would result in missing individual and group sessions. Examples of ED-specific TIBs include being unable to concentrate or remember discussions in session due to malnourishment, unable to participate effectively in skills groups due to being hyper-focused on food or weight concerns, or missing treatment due to hospitalizations for medical instability.

"Noncollaborative behaviors" refer to verbal and nonverbal indicators that a client is not able to work from a collaborative, open, or willing stance. Common DBT examples include not talking in session or arguing constantly about the treatment approach. ED-specific behaviors might include continually arguing about the need to monitor labs, exercising against medical advice, water loading before being weighed, lying about pill use (e.g., laxatives/diet pills/diuretics), not bringing enough food to a planned exposure, hiding food in the office, or not being truthful on the MED-DBT diary cards.

"Noncompliant behaviors" refer to a lack of engagement in planned, expected, or necessary treatment tasks such as completing skills homework or not calling for phone coaching when suicidal. Examples of ED-specific behaviors include not getting labs and vitals done in the service of addressing a T1, refusing to see a medical provider, not filling out/partially completing MED-DBT diary cards, not engaging in planned food or weight exposures, or refusing to practice DBT skills when experiencing urges to binge or purge.

### Category 2: Behaviors That Interfere with Other Clients

Creating safe spaces for all clients is necessary, and we expect our clients to engage appropriately with one another in the service of contributing to safety. Behaviors that would be considered therapy-interfering in this respect include those that are overtly critical, oppressive, discriminatory, damaging, and hostile. ED-specific examples include comparing body weights, recommending pro-anorexia media accounts to co-patients, making fat-phobic or weight-biased comments, repeatedly checking wrist or waist circumference or feeling for bones in group settings. While it is important to remember that one of the interpersonal goals of MED-DBT is to help our clients manage conflict and polarization more effectively, hostile and discriminatory behaviors must be actively and quickly targeted.

### Category 3: Behaviors That Burn Out Therapists or Push Organizational Limits

With pervasive emotional and interpersonal difficulties, unstable eating patterns, and having adapted to chronically invalidating environments, our clients will engage in behaviors that push our limits (and we will engage in behaviors that push theirs!). Linehan teaches that DBT therapists are transparent with their clients with respect to what burns them out and that it is a goal of the treatment to help clients engage in ways that don't push caring others away. While it may be challenging to name and target these things, avoiding them leads to non-adherent treatment, premature termination of treatment, patient blaming, and/or hanging onto clients for years even though they are not getting better. It is also our experience that treatment is not effective when practitioners are burnt out, feel resentful, or believe they are ineffective. For these reasons, MED-DBT is proactive around burnout. This means we observe and describe our limits directly with clients from the beginning of treatment and as they come up over the course of the therapy. By doing so, we collaboratively aim to prevent therapist burnout and model healthy communication with our clients. These TIBs can be categorized as those that push the therapist's limit, push organizational limits, and those that reduce therapist motivation.

We all have limits. Limits are an important part of self-awareness and essential to healthy relationships. Our limits are not fixed or static; rather, they ebb and flow and change over time and context. You may notice that certain behaviors always push your limits while others only become problematic for you under certain circumstances. In addition to the behaviors Linehan (1993) and Chapman and Rosenthal (2015) outline in standard DBT, we have observed behaviors specific to EDs that tend to push therapist limits. These include, but are not limited to the following:

- Continuing to lose weight while underweight or when medically unstable
- Refusing to collaborate on weight goals
- Refusing medical advice
- Engaging in ED behaviors while pregnant
- Receiving multiple phone coaching calls per day for each meal and snack
- Becoming angry or shutting down when the therapist does only brief phone coaching for a meal instead of talking about therapy topics between sessions
- Receiving critical or hostile emails from a client's family who wants to know why more weight gain hasn't happened
- Not accepting medical instability criteria
- Asking the therapist to lie to the doctor about their symptom/behaviors
- Prioritizing therapy with other non-MED-DBT providers who are giving contradictory recommendations around food, weight, and EDs
- Demanding more support around meals/snacks or weight than the therapist can provide

Some examples of behaviors that push organizational limits are as follows:

- Vomiting in the lobby restroom causing tension with the landlord
- Having two treating dietitians or two ED psychiatrists
- BMI dropping below a clinic's cutoff requiring a higher level of care
- Engaging in exercise in the waiting room

Lastly, behaviors that decrease the therapist's motivation include the following:

- Slow ED progress
- Lying about food and fluid intake
- Unwilling to talk with their doctor about getting labs/vitals
- Unwilling to talk about ED symptoms

How do Jules's symptoms fit? Jules presents with several T2 behaviors, including the following:

- Taking potassium supplements before labs to influence results
- Stating that they do not want to work on the ED
- Stating that they do not view the ED as serious
- Living an hour away from the clinic and being unable to drive
- Wanting to focus solely on PTSD
- Expressing anger when providers have requested to focus on non-trauma-related symptoms
- Stating that they are wary of MED-DBT given that DBT skills didn't work in the past
- Decreased trust in your ability to provide a safe and affirmative environment

It is unclear whether the substance use described by Jules is therapy-interfering. It may or may not be if they are able to attend, be alert, and demonstrate that it does not interfere (Dimeff et al., 2021). Given that Jules recently lost 35 pounds, it is also unclear whether they are continuing to lose weight. While continued weight loss is not always T2, in this case it would be treatment-interfering in the context of their medical instability and would be targeted as such until the medical instability is resolved.

## TIBs of MED-DBT Clinicians

MED-DBT therapists are mindful of, openly discuss, and actively target their own treatment-interfering behaviors. We commit to maintaining an open, flexible, and non-defensive stance with respect to addressing and correcting our own TIBs. We expect them to happen and hold ourselves to the same standard with which we hold our clients when it comes to addressing the things that get in the way of conducting or engaging with the treatment. Without attention to how the provider is engaging in TIBs, we run the risk of focusing solely on what the client is or is not doing when things get challenging instead of exploring the transactions between the therapist and the client that cause difficulties.

In MED-DBT, we observe and target the same therapist-interfering behaviors as one does in standard DBT (Linehan, 1993; Chapman & Rosenthal, 2015). However, there are distinctive ways therapist TIBs show up when treating EDs. As Linehan described, our own emotions, conflict management skills, and tolerance of uncertainty can become therapy-interfering: "Attempts to ameliorate patient suffering often lead to reinforcements of dysfunctional behaviors, which, rather than reducing suffering, actually increase it in the long run" (Linehan, 1993, p. 139). This is all too familiar when working with our multidiagnostic clients. Practitioners often experience fear or frustration when managing medical and nutritional issues and have difficulty tolerating the distress our clients experience. This can mean that important limits are not upheld or that arbitrary and punitive limits are implemented for reasons that usually soothe the client, the family, or the therapist in the short term but don't lead to LWL changes in the long run.

There are also unique circumstances related to weight, shape, and eating that can arise in this model that can be very interfering. We all have personal experiences with body weight and nutrition and have, therefore, developed attitudes, biases, and behaviors with respect to these areas in our own lives. For example, most of us have grown up immersed in diet culture. If we are not mindful or active in learning about, identifying, and addressing our own weight biases, relationship to diet culture, and beliefs about what constitutes "healthy" eating, we may engage in invalidating behaviors or offer treatment decisions that are not in the best interest of our clients. Without adequate training and supervision, therapists may make suggestions that "worked for them" (e.g., a therapist recommending a low-carb diet and not eating after 8:00 P.M. to a client with AN-R) without realizing how inappropriate this is for the client.

## Oriented to Change versus Acceptance

In an effort to provide you with a guide, we have expanded Linehan's work on therapeutic imbalances to include MED-DBT-specific examples. Just as Linehan recognized that relying solely on behaviorism to treat patients with BPD was ineffective, emphasizing change-based ED interventions as the primary mode of action is also not sufficient for our clients who require a more dialectical approach. Examples of being imbalanced with change-based strategies in ED treatment include the following:

- Relying solely on CBT interventions rather than using dialectic strategies
- Predominantly pushing for T3 meal plan compliance versus targeting suicidal behavior
- Defining progress solely based on weight or eating
- Assuming all clients can eat all foods in a certain manner, or within certain time frames despite oral sensitivities or without accounting for co-occurring diagnoses
- Expecting clients to engage in mindfulness practices that rely on interoceptive awareness
- Consults with the team rather than to the patient (e.g., talks to the dietitian on behalf of the patient instead of helping the patient build skills to communicate directly with the dietitian)
- Focusing solely on "full recovery" as the goal of treatment

On the other hand, if you focus too heavily on acceptance-based strategies, you may find that your clients enjoy talking with you but their behaviors do not improve. We have observed that, for our clients, acceptance-based or purely supportive therapy approaches can lead to increased hopelessness and a worsening of ED and suicidal behaviors over time and sometimes anger at the therapist that nothing is working. Examples of being imbalanced with acceptance-based strategies include the following:

- Validating how hard it is to eat without pushing for change
- Not problem solving when your client does not get lab work done
- Prioritizing talking about the client's agenda without doing a chain analysis on targeted ED behaviors
- Reinforcing a client's nonattendance in group because they were not feeling well
- Setting treatment goals too low or not setting them at all

As you read through these examples, we encourage you to identify where you see yourself in each of the identified domains. What would you need to work on in order to find more of a balance between these two approaches?

### Compassionate Flexibility versus Unwavering Centeredness

When working with our clients, it is not uncommon for clinicians to oscillate between excessive flexibility and rigidly held patterns of responding to client behavior. For example, therapists may abandon or modify evidence-based protocols when they are challenged, burned out, or as a way to reduce crisis behaviors. Flexibility is important *and* excessive flexibility may reinforce the very behaviors we need to help our clients change if we are to achieve an LWL. Examples of excessive flexibility include the following:

- Stopping MED-DBT when things become challenging
- Abandoning the target hierarchy because the client doesn't want to talk about T1 behaviors
- Not expecting a client to complete the MED-DBT diary card because they felt it was too upsetting
- Extending the therapy hour when the client arrives late
- Constantly reorganizing sessions and skills attendance to accommodate medical and dietitian appointments

On the other hand, though there are times that call for a therapist's unwavering centeredness to the model, rigidly held positions are rarely effective for our clients. Examples of rigidly held positions include the following:

- Insisting on using the same DBT skills during a meal when they haven't been beneficial

- Rigidly reviewing the food log when your client is in an emotional crisis
- Hanging on to a client when the treatment is not working
- Maintaining narrow or binary views of recovery (e.g., must achieve a certain weight)

Again, where do you see yourself on the continuum between excessive flexibility and rigidity? What would you need to work on in order to find more of a balance between these two approaches?

## Nurturing versus Demanding Change

A patient we treated with AN-BP and chronic suicidality in the context of a sexual abuse history had been in and out of ED programs for years with little success. In our assessment phase with the client, we observed that her previous providers tended to either take a very benevolent role (e.g., treating her as fragile, unable to make decisions, and approaching her as excessively vulnerable) or a very demanding role in which she was expected to solve her own problems and act in ways that far exceeded her capacities. It is also common for providers to oscillate between these two positions. While we need to help our clients learn to better manage their symptoms and environments, treating them as incapable and/or demanding behaviors that exceed their capacities is treatment-interfering. The MED-DBT therapist stays mindful of this and works to do what is effective for the client, not what is easiest for them.

Some examples of getting stuck in a nurturing frame include the following:

- Treating your client as overly fragile, not holding them to treatment requirements
- Assuming your client is incompetent or unable to contribute to treatment planning due to low body weight
- Treating your client as if they are unable to tolerate change
- Not offering pretreatment to a potential client due to significant food restriction
- Intense anxiety about a client's medical stability that leads to avoidance of using the target hierarchy

- Not addressing ED issues as part of treatment so as not to upset the client

And some examples of getting stuck in a demanding change frame are as follows:

- Demanding that your client be weighed (without discussion) when they have expressed concern about the practice
- "You are going to die" communications
- Requiring your client to eat feared foods in the absence of distress tolerance skills
- Focusing on changing ED thoughts without attending to emotion regulation
- Abruptly discharging your client when progress is slow
- Assuming that patients should be better able to regulate emotions

## Reciprocal versus Irreverent Communication

Therapists can also find themselves getting stuck in their communication styles. Reciprocal communication in DBT is an acceptance-based strategy aimed at enhancing the therapeutic relationship. It refers to a responsive, warm, affectionate, and genuine stance that emphasizes equality between client and therapist. Irreverent communication (mentioned in Chapter 9) is a change-based technique in which the therapist adopts a playful, humorous, flippant, unusual, and/or direct style to keep the client slightly off balance. For instance, a client in pretreatment told her therapist that she planned to return to university so she could "keep" her anorexia and lose the weight she was forced to gain in a higher level of care. The therapist replied in a way the client was not expecting: "Oh, shoot. I didn't realize you already had this all figured out. I guess you don't need me, then?" Problems arise when therapists rely on one type of communication over the other. MED-DBT requires clinicians to be strategic in their communication styles and to use a style that is effective for the situation at hand, not the one that comes most naturally to them.

Some examples of getting stuck in reciprocal communication would be if a therapist is always warm when the client does not complete required tasks (e.g., lab work, diary card), consistently communicates affection when the client is not willing to talk about poor concentration during sessions due to malnourishment, or does not directly confront T1 or T2 ED behaviors. Examples of getting stuck in irreverent communication include: A therapist overly relies on humor when a more genuine stance was needed, their use of flippant communication around ED thoughts minimizes the impact of diet culture for the client/perpetuates invalidation, or irreverence is used without balancing reciprocal communication.

## Behaviors Showing Lack of Respect for the Client

MED-DBT is predicated on a deep respect for, and efforts to establish equality between, you and your client. Therefore, any behavior that communicates (verbally or nonverbally) a lack of respect for your client would be addressed as a T2 behavior. Examples include the following:

- Communicating/modeling fat-phobic, weight-biased beliefs
- The therapist's own ED behaviors interfere (e.g., unwillingness to eat the same food as the client during meals, getting triggered by the client's ED and not addressing it in the consult team, being undernourished leading to poor concentration in session)
- Not consulting with the client about treatment planning, assuming the expert role
- Breaking confidentiality and disclosing ED behaviors to the client's family
- Beliefs or statements that assume clients in smaller bodies are more deserving of care or are experiencing more severe illness than clients in larger bodies reflect weight bias and would be addressed as T2 behaviors
- Emphasizing cisgendered or White body narratives for 2SLGBTQ+ clients
- Labeling clients as treatment resistant, attention-seeking, or hostile
- Not adequately trained (or outdated training) in ED theory and treatment
- Trying to deliver MED-DBT without adequate training or supervision
- Being unprepared for/lacking training in conducting therapeutic meals
- Making treatment decisions for your client, not with your client (e.g., choosing CBT-ED for them and not offering/educating about MED-DBT)

## Target 3: Quality-of-Life-Interfering Behaviors

The final priority on the target hierarchy is reserved for behaviors that interfere with one's ability to build an LWL. In standard DBT, this often includes substance use difficulties, relationship problems, employment/school challenges, and housing issues that are not T1 or T2. In MED-DBT, this applies to ED behaviors that are not imminently life-threatening or actively therapy-interfering. This is a significant shift from traditional ED approaches that translates into learning to tolerate a slower pace of change or not imposing your desire to ameliorate all of a client's ED behaviors. The challenge is that our clients (and their families) often want us to focus here (on quality-of-life-interfering behaviors) without adequately addressing and building skills to reduce the T1 and T2 behaviors that ultimately become barriers to quality of life.

How do Jules's symptoms fit with this? Jules wants very much to focus on PTSD. In the target hierarchy, we would do so once there has been a sustained period of no T1 behaviors and a reduction in T2 behaviors, allowing space to target the things that impact their quality of life. According to Melanie Harned's DBT-PE (dialectical behavior therapy—prolonged exposure) protocol, it is recommended that clients have a period of 3 months of no T1 behaviors before moving into focused trauma work. This is not designed to be punitive, but rather to radically accept that most clients are unable to effectively manage intense trauma work concurrently with T1 symptoms (Harned, 2022).

Jules's substance use likely interferes with their quality of life, and it is important not to make assumptions. As noted earlier, the substance use that triggers suicide and self-injury would be the T1 behavior, while other substance use would not. We would collaborate and discuss with Jules regarding the function of using cannabis daily and their use of cocaine in the context of their LWL goals and targets from that perspective. Other potential T3 targets for Jules might include relationship issues, school or work challenges, body image disturbance, or eating with friends and family.

Review the case study on Jules that was presented at the start of this chapter. Try to identify the thoughts, emotions, and behaviors you might experience when sitting across from Jules who is expressing doubt in your model, a strong desire to direct the treatment toward PTSD, feelings of anger toward past providers, and does not see the ED as a primary focus. Where might you get unbalanced?

## Summary

The target hierarchy is the "blueprint" or pathway for how to build an LWL. The hierarchy is not imposed; rather, it is a shared agreement between you and your client. Building an LWL requires clients to stay alive while they work with you, which means they must be willing to target imminently life-threatening ED symptoms in addition to suicide and self-injury. MED-DBT will not be effective if our clients cannot receive a full course of treatment, therefore client and therapist agree to target anything that compromises engagement. Finally, building an LWL means addressing the things that interfere with quality of life. The hierarchy is used to set the agenda for each session and create structure amid chaos in order to help your client reach their goals.

With the target hierarchy in place, you and your client now have a shared roadmap to guide your work together. The next step is translating that hierarchy into action—session by session. In the following chapter, we walk through how to structure and deliver individual MED-DBT therapy, the central modality where targets are addressed, progress is tracked, and meaningful change begins.

# PART IV
# THE MED-DBT PROTOCOL

This part of the book outlines how to deliver MED-DBT in practice. Now that you've established the theoretical framework and completed the pre-treatment phase, this section walks you through the core treatment components of the model. Each chapter offers practical guidance on structuring sessions, using diary cards effectively, conducting chain and missing links analyses, teaching skills with nuance, offering phone coaching, and applying contingency management strategies. We also highlight the essential role of the consultation team in maintaining treatment fidelity and therapist sustainability. Finally, we conclude with a chapter on how to navigate endings and treatment transitions with clarity and compassion.

This part of the book includes the following:

- Chapter 12: Individual Session Structure
- Chapter 13: MED-DBT Diary Cards
- Chapter 14: Behavior-Chain and Missing Links Analysis
- Chapter 15: Considerations for Teaching DBT Skills
- Chapter 16: Adaptations for Phone Coaching
- Chapter 17: Contingency Management in DBT
- Chapter 18: Consult Teams in MED-DBT
- Chapter 19: Transitions and Ending Well

# 12

# Individual Session Structure

Now that the pretreatment phase is complete and you and your client agree that MED-DBT is a good fit, comprehensive treatment begins. At this time, you will enroll your client in a MED-DBT skills group (Chapter 15), begin phone coaching (Chapter 16), and start weekly individual MED-DBT therapy sessions. Your client will need help getting used to MED-DBT sessions and acclimating to the multimodal nature of the treatment, and you will need support from your team to stay adherent (see Chapter 18).

The individual therapist is the primary provider of the MED-DBT treatment. Together with your client, you form the main "hub" of the model, directing the treatment targets, developing treatment plans, coordinating as needed with other care providers (e.g., physicians, dietitians), and evaluating progress. We receive many questions about what exactly an individual MED-DBT session looks like. Given that our treatment is principle-driven, not protocol-driven, sessions don't all look alike. That said, we will offer some general guidelines that define most MED-DBT individual therapy sessions.

MED-DBT individual sessions involve the same structure that Linehan outlined in her 1993 text. We assume that you are familiar with standard DBT sessions (both in terms of structure and strategy) and that you have a sound understanding of the therapeutic tasks that define those individual sessions. We do not describe standard DBT session strategies in this chapter; rather, we provide an overview of MED-DBT sessions with emphasis on how they differ or require adaptation.

## The "What" of Individual Sessions

We have divided individual session guidelines into a set of "what" and "how" recommendations. Some of the "what" strategies have been described in other chapters (e.g., target hierarchy, chain analysis) and are not repeated in this section.

### Setting Up Your Space

We feel strongly that it is our job in the ED field to ensure spaces that are weight-inclusive and free of diet culture. You might be surprised to learn about all the ways weight bias shows up in the healthcare setting. From chairs and medical equipment that only work for smaller body sizes to images, magazines, and art that promote thin, cisgender, and Western body ideals, we encourage you to take time to reflect on whether your clinical working spaces (virtual or otherwise) demonstrate your commitment to an inclusive and safe place for all body shapes and sizes. This is especially important with skills group rooms that often have smaller chairs around a table that may not be appropriate for clients in larger bodies. Your space is an extension of your values and beliefs, and reflects your anti-diet, anti-oppressive, and weight-inclusive views.

### Beginning the Session: Setting the Agenda

The first part of your session is used to gather the information needed to set the agenda. You will work with your client to accomplish the following early session tasks:

- Welcome/reinforce your client for attending the session. While it sounds obvious, it is important to communicate that you are glad your client chose to attend the appointment. This is especially relevant when your client may be in crisis or tends to cope by avoiding. A warm, genuine welcome is both validating and reinforcing of effective behavior.
- Weight check if part of your treatment plan. Those trained in standard DBT probably don't have scales in their office and may feel quite uncomfortable with the idea of weighing a client. On the other hand, our CBT-ED and FBT colleagues weigh patients weekly as a central part of those evidence-based treatments. In MED-DBT, we maintain

a dialectical stance and seek to measure our client's weights when it is collaborative and necessary in order to resolve a targeted behavior. We do not weigh patients "just because" they have an ED. Conversations about weighing a patient must involve the pros and cons of being weighed, a rationale for how it connects to the target hierarchy, and the freedom to choose not to be weighed. Additionally, these conversations must include a focus on how being weighed or not may have been invalidating in the past for our clients. When regularly weighing a client is mandated as a condition of the treatment, we (1) cannot have informed consent and (2) are no longer acting dialectically. We *may* weigh a client in MED-DBT (with consent) when

- ☐ A client is losing weight and approaching a riskier zone in terms of medical stability (e.g., your client is nearing a weight range that has historically led to bradycardia and hospital admission).
- ☐ A client insists on not being weighed or knowing their weight, and their weight steadily increases and eventually becomes an issue.
- ☐ You are working toward a weight gain goal and need to track progress.
- ☐ The sight of one's weight leads to suicidal behavior, and you agree that exposure may help.
- ☐ Fears about weight gain interfere with the client's ability to adequately feed themselves (e.g., avoiding foods or food groups due to a fear of weight changes).
- ☐ Monitoring and discussing weight fluctuations/patterns might help to reduce distressing thoughts through habituation.
- ☐ Working to decrease obsessive weighing that some clients engage in between sessions (e.g., being weighed only in the therapist's office once a week can be helpful).

As we have outlined, the overarching goal of MED-DBT is not necessarily weight gain (unless it is related to a T1 or T2 situation). Rather, the goal is to build a life that your client wants to live. Tracking body weight is not always needed in order to achieve this. In fact, not being weighed can be protective for some clients with histories of fat-shaming and weight discrimination. It is essential that you have training in weight bias in order to ensure that assumptions are not being made about a client, their body weight, or their responses to the possibility of being weighed.

If you are weighing your client, discuss ahead of time how weight will be taken, whether you will use a blind weight (e.g., where the client does not see/know their weight) or a non-blind weight, how weight will be tracked and used to inform the session, and for how long your client will need to be weighed. There should be regular and collaborative evaluation regarding the effectiveness of the weighing intervention. We recommend weighing clients at the start of your appointment both to inform the session agenda and to ensure adequate time to manage emotions and thoughts that may arise related to the weight check.

- *Review diary cards.* As in standard DBT, diary cards are reviewed out loud at the start of each session and in a manner that conveys their importance. As will be discussed in Chapter 13, MED-DBT diary cards are more involved than standard diary cards: In addition to suicide attempts and self-injury, they include food and fluid intake and ED urges and behaviors. You want to have enough time to scan each card for relevant data in order to set the agenda but not spend so much time that the bulk of the session is focused on them. Your client is asked to help point out important targets while you both review diary cards. If your client does not have a diary card completed, that is added to your session agenda as a T2 behavior. Depending on your case conceptualization, you might spend session time completing a missing link analysis or helping your client to complete their diary cards.
- *Establish the session agenda.* Work with your client to set the agenda for the session by determining where their behaviors fall on the target hierarchy. As discussed in Chapter 7, T1 behaviors are prioritized, followed by T2, then T3. That said, be open to negotiating the agenda to accommodate things the client wants to address without losing sight of the target hierarchy. For instance, you may agree to carve out time (10 minutes) to discuss a job opportunity (T3) while also ensuring time to talk about bradycardia (T1, 20 minutes) and missing the last physician appointment (T2, 15 minutes). Linking to prior commitments can also be helpful when clients don't want to talk about T1 or T2 behaviors (e.g., "I know one of the things you didn't like about other treatments is that you felt there was no clear direction. You thought the hierarchy was a decent way to move forward; is that still true?"). Alternatively, you might add "disagreement about the target hierarchy" to the session agenda as a T2 behavior to be discussed.

## Case Study: Olivia

Olivia arrived at our program in a very anxious state. She had tried multiple standard ED treatments and was never able to last more than a few weeks. She shook as she reported her history during the assessment. She was bradycardic and restricting food and fluid intake most days. We talked about the pros and cons of getting a baseline weight, which she was agreeable to, until she walked into the weight room. She backed up against the wall and shook more. We stopped and spent several weeks trying to better understand what she was experiencing and the level of intense emotionality. Eventually, she disclosed that part of her sexual trauma history involved being weighed by her abuser.

We share this account because it is easy to make assumptions about why someone doesn't want to be weighed or to assume that just because a person has an ED, they "should" be weighed and in a particular manner. For Olivia, not only was she confronting the ED every time she was asked to be weighed, but she was also in a full-blown trauma exposure. Olivia's disclosure allowed us to deeply validate her pain and arrive at a synthesis in which we worked on distress tolerance skills first for grounding and then a graded exposure hierarchy to be weighed, all with her consent and feedback about the process along the way.

## Continuing the Agenda

- Follow up on homework and check in on skills group engagement. Homework that is not followed up on is unlikely to be completed or viewed as valuable. It is also often the case that therapists forget to ask about homework (T2); therefore, you might want to have a standing event on the agenda to make sure homework gets discussed!
- The bulk of your sessions will focus on exploring how symptoms arise and are maintained while collaboratively generating solutions to try for homework. Thus, most MED-DBT sessions will include a behavior-chain or missing link analysis and a solution analysis (it is rare for an individual session not to include one of these interventions). These highly exploratory tools (discussed fully in Chapter 13) shed light on details and nuances related to why a behavior happens over and over again even though it is ruining your client's life. Acting like two detectives, you and your client enter into a space of collaborative curiosity designed to empower and elevate both of you to a more accurate

understanding of a behavior. This process leads to a brainstorming session and a coactive generation of ideas to circumvent or overcome old ways of coping.

- Session-ending strategies. Leave time in your sessions to summarize, set a homework plan, evaluate what might get in the way of the homework. Some clients respond well to a brief wind-down at the end of the session. MED-DBT sessions are busy and can feel intense, especially when your client is malnourished and emotionally vulnerable. Writing down homework and key takeaways can help when memory or attentional issues arise.

## Can My Client's Doctor or Dietitian Weigh Them/Review Food Intake Instead of Me?

MED-DBT is principle-driven, so decisions about who and how your client monitors their weight need to be in line with the philosophy and goals of the treatment. Having someone outside of your team manage weight and nutrition review with your client may be fine or it may be therapy-interfering. In general, our preference is for you to manage those treatment pieces in the context of the individual therapy sessions for the following reasons:

1. Many physicians and dietitians are not ED-trained and may miss or misinterpret data or may not track in a timely manner.
2. Communication issues tend to arise. Outside providers do not participate in your MED-DBT consult team, and it can be difficult to ensure appropriate and timely access to the data they are collecting.
3. Inaccurate, late, or poor communication will make it very difficult to set an effective agenda in your therapy session. For example, if monitoring weight is related to a T1 behavior (e.g., bradycardia), you would need to know the weight data at the start of your weekly session in order to know whether and where it sits on the target hierarchy. Another example would be trying to help your client eat in high-stress situations but not having a full review of their intake over the week to inform the session and your approach.
4. Working with your client to manage weight and eating gives you the opportunity to model MED-DBT theory and philosophy. For example, you might approach weight loss dialectically and irreverently or use a missing link analysis to better understand why restriction happens at breakfast before jumping to solutions. Linking weight loss or ED

symptoms to your client's life worth living goals is another example of helping your client activate their wise mind (e.g., "I know you want to travel in the spring, and I wonder how this recent weight loss helps or delays that plan").

Sometimes if we determine that an outside provider can monitor weight and food intake, we attend to whether and when it becomes treatment-interfering and generate solutions with our client. It is important for them to learn to manage their network of providers, and this could present an opportunity for them to do that effectively.

## The "How" of Individual Sessions

The "what" recommendations we have outlined, while necessary, are not sufficient to deliver an adherent MED-DBT individual session. As a MED-DBT therapist, you will demonstrate the theories, assumptions, and team agreements through words and actions, model a dialectical and weight-inclusive worldview, stay mindful of the ways you can become unbalanced, and use the range of DBT stylistic and commitment strategies as needed. Sessions are dynamic and exemplify the "movement, speed, and flow" that Linehan described as a key feature of any DBT work (1993). The following list serves as a reminder regarding the strategies used in MED-DBT sessions. We recommend using the DBT Adherence & Fidelity Project's website (*www.dbtadherence.com*) to review these in-session therapist tasks in detail:

- Maintain an emotion focus
- Model dialectical thinking/use dialectical strategies
- Use irreverence and reciprocal communication strategies
- Use levels of validation
- Weave in commitment strategies
- Link to the adapted biosocial theory
- Use contingency management/learning theory
- Observe limits
- Apply cognitive modification
- Focus on formal or informal exposure strategies
- Generate solutions

Although your clients get a sense of you and of MED-DBT in the pretreatment phase, getting used to the structure and tasks of individual sessions can take time. Managing crises and treatment-interfering behaviors typically dominate early sessions. Much like a plane trying to take off in stormy weather, it is important for you and your client to anticipate the turbulence. Sometimes therapists expect their clients to be fully engaged once the pretreatment phase is complete. In our experience, this is not the case! In fact, the work for both client and therapist tends to intensify once pretreatment has ended and therapy begins. This is usually a highly emotional and vulnerable time for our clients (and sometimes the therapists!). Our clients want help, they think the model makes sense *and* they still want to stay safe and hang onto habitual ways of coping. It is important to remember that our clients have experienced different therapy modalities and unique environments that have responded in specific ways to their symptoms. Your client may expect you to respond in similar ways and may find it challenging at first when you interact differently to their modes of coping.

For example, a client may find it uncomfortable when you do a missing link analysis when they did not complete their food logs and when previous therapists did not address this behavior. Other clients may expect you to respond in particular ways when they are medically unstable, suicidal, or losing weight. The unique and transactional manner in which MED-DBT therapists conduct themselves is often experienced as refreshing *and* difficult for clients.

## Family Meetings/Sessions

While the adolescent MED-DBT model includes regular family involvement (e.g., multifamily skills groups, parent coaching), the adult MED-DBT model does not mandate that families must be involved. Nonetheless, issues around when to involve the family do arise fairly frequently with our adult clients. For example, parents of young adults who are living at home and are dependent on them for food/eating and emotional support often need help. It is a challenging dialectic: Excluding parents is rarely effective *and* adult clients have legal rights to their privacy. This can prove to be a difficult and treatment-interfering issue when your client is not doing well, is unwilling to involve their parents, and the family is demanding answers. These T2 issues are added to your individual session agenda until they are resolved.

We highlight this tension with our clients in order to help them make wise-mind decisions (e.g., "Yes, you have the right not to involve your parents, and also the less they know, the more they hover over you and feel anxious"). Sometimes, when parents are calling and feeling anxious or confused about their loved one's treatment plan and we don't have the client's permission to speak about their care, we invite parents to meet with another member of the MED-DBT team to provide support. In other instances, we have had parents join a different DBT skills group so they can learn the philosophy and strategies themselves. In these cases, your team must be vigilant not to share confidential information.

### Offering Additional Sessions to Address Co-Occurring Issues?

In general, we do not recommend adding additional therapy sessions, mostly because our clients already have a significant amount of work to do with respect to managing T1 and T2 behaviors and keeping up with skills homework. There may be circumstances, however, when a co-occurring condition is interfering and might respond to additional sessions that provide evidence-based treatment. For example, say your client has anorexia and severe OCD. The bidirectional nature of these two illnesses has made efforts to stabilize their health almost impossible (e.g., severe rituals around eating and dressing that have interfered with your client's ability to increase food intake at all). You might consider offering concurrent OCD treatment with another member of the MED-DBT team. In these cases, the OCD sessions would follow a CBT/ERP protocol and only be used to focus on OCD (and not to discuss other client needs, which would remain with the primary individual therapist).

## Summary

Like in standard DBT, MED-DBT therapists use the principles and theories of DBT to determine how to organize each session. When overwhelmed or stuck, guidance from the team provides direction on an as-needed basis. With many symptoms presenting in a given week and only a 50-minute session to work with, the therapist and client must work together to stay focused and effective. Most sessions will include a review of the diary cards, agenda setting, and a behavior chain/missing links analysis of targeted behaviors (discussed in Chapter 13) with a corresponding solution analysis. But before you can collaboratively set an agenda or effectively analyze behavior, you need accurate, real-time information about what's happening between sessions. The next chapter introduces the MED-DBT diary card—a foundational tool for tracking patterns, identifying treatment targets, and helping clients build insight into the relationship between their emotions, behaviors, and symptoms. You'll also learn how to navigate common challenges clients may have with tracking, especially in the context of EDs.

# 13

# MED-DBT Diary Cards

When Cara started MED-DBT, she presented with chronic suicidal ideation, frequent cutting, excessive exercise, restrained eating, and purging behaviors. She felt intense and daily body image disturbance and could identify disgust and fear but, when prompted, she stated that she "had no idea" what else she was feeling. She was vague about what she ate and noted periods in her life where she either obsessed about intake or "paid no attention whatsoever." Cara had difficulty identifying how often her symptoms occurred other than with qualifiers such as "always" or "sometimes" and usually a shrug of the shoulders. She wasn't sure whether thoughts of suicide or self-injury were connected to ED symptoms or vice versa and felt that there was no pattern to how her thoughts, urges, and behaviors happened. She didn't like the idea of doing a daily diary card and said that food monitoring in the past only made her ED symptoms worse.

Tracking symptoms is not new to DBT or to mainstream ED approaches. While the former focuses on monitoring suicidal and self-injurious behaviors, emotions, and DBT skill use, the latter typically requires clients to track food and fluid intake. One of the difficulties we faced in developing MED-DBT was the absence of a diary card that tracked *both* DBT and ED targets together. Thus, this chapter outlines our adapted DBT diary cards and how to use them with your clients.

## Setting the Stage

### Step 1: Familiarize Yourself with the MED-DBT Diary Card

MED-DBT diary cards can be overwhelming to learn and use effectively. To help you build competence in using and teaching clients how to use them, we recommend that you practice tracking your own food and fluid intake, emotions, and other behaviors ahead of asking your client to do so. Clinicians have shared with us that completing their own MED-DBT diary cards was more challenging than they anticipated. Some reported difficulty remembering to record meals and snacks, accurately tracking intake or sensing hunger and fullness cues, and others reported anxiety or shame writing down their eating habits. Practicing helps you anticipate obstacles to using diary cards and increases compassion for your clients as they will struggle in similar ways.

## Step 2: Build and Maintain Commitment to Using Diary Cards

Clients in MED-DBT complete diary cards on a daily basis, tracking targeted ED behaviors in addition to suicide, self-injury, emotions, and skills. This can be a big ask for you and your client! Keep in mind that MED-DBT diary cards produce more data than standard DBT diary cards. Since we collect food/fluid intake daily, there are seven pages to review each week (in addition to one page that covers skill use during the week). Keeping an eye on your client's commitment and your own motivation to use diary cards is an important treatment task. Discussing and revisiting the following rationale for using diary cards is one way to reinforce their use:

- Diary cards are meant to be a mindful practice, meaning that the aim is to use the mindfulness "what" and "how" skills in this context. As Cara reported in our case study at the start of this chapter, making connections between ED behaviors, emotions, and suicide was difficult. She was unsure whether there was a relationship between various thoughts and behaviors. She also described concerns that tracking would make her ED worse. Diary cards can help to support a practice of observing, describing, and talking about food intake with curiosity and non-judgment.
- Diary cards are designed to help you and your client find a synthesis between compulsively counting calories/focusing excessively on food and complete avoidance of food talk/planning. This means that you and your client will have ongoing discussions about exactly how much food/fluid information is needed and what is effective (rather than being rigid) at different times over the course of treatment. For example, if your client is losing weight and they don't know why, getting precise

details will matter. On the other hand, if your client is overcontrolled and gets lost in the details of tracking perfectly so that it interferes with treatment goals, you might opt for less detail.

- Diary cards are the fastest way to communicate large amounts of information. When there is so much going on (e.g., suicidal thinking, self-injury, restriction, binge eating, purging, laxative abuse, etc.), it would take most of the session just to get caught up on the details of the preceding week. Using diary cards means key details can be communicated quickly, allowing more time in session to work on building an LWL.
- Diary cards aid in more precise recall. It is very difficult to remember what one ate last week, how intense an urge to purge was five days ago, or what one's hunger and fullness cues were in retrospect. You and your client will be better equipped to understand cycles and patterns and develop effective treatment plans with accurate data. Accuracy also helps to minimize misunderstandings.
- Diary cards are empowering in that they usually provide missing data that can be used to better support LWL goals. The diary card points you and your client in helpful directions and is used to organize session time to maximize progress.

### Step 3: Filling Out a Diary Card with Your Client

As stated, it is your job to stay dialectical and approach the tracking of food/fluid and other symptoms in a way that is effective and not just arbitrary (i.e., you have an ED therefore you must track everything all the time). That said, it is important to never lose sight of the eating disorder as relapses often begin with very subtle shifts in eating patterns.

Successful implementation of the diary card starts with a thorough explanation and demonstration of its use with your client. A simple explanation without demonstration is not sufficient. We suggest working through a diary card with your client using symptoms, urges, and behaviors from the previous day as an example. Explain that the diary card comes in two parts:

- Part A tracks food and fluid intake, ED and suicidal urges and behaviors, and includes a section on rating emotions. (Part A is used by your client *every day;* therefore, your client receives *seven copies of Part A per week.*)
- Part B tracks use of DBT and ED skills and strategies. Your client receives *one copy of Part B per week.*

In preparation, have diary cards printed out for in-person sessions or uploaded onto your computer for virtual sessions. At the end of this chapter, we include a MED-DBT diary card (Handout 13.1) to use with your clients. Also ensure your client has access to Handout 13.2, How to Use MED-DBT Diary Cards, at the end of this chapter.

## Part A: The Details

Let's walk through the columns on Handout 13.1 from left to right.

### Time of Day

It is important for your client to track *when* they ate and consumed fluids. This helps you detect restrictive or delayed patterns of eating (e.g., going longer than 3 hours without food). The time-of-day column can also be used to facilitate mechanical eating (or by-the-clock eating) by prepopulating the times that your client is scheduled to eat.

### Meals/Food Intake

In this section, your client can write down what they ate during the day. The level of detail is determined by your conceptualization of the client (using the biosocial theory) and the specific treatment targets (per the hierarchy). Let's go over a few potential scenarios to help clarify.

*Scenario 1:* Your client is medically unstable, has lost 2 pounds in the last week, has difficulty understanding why this is happening because they report eating three meals and two snacks each day with no ED behaviors (e.g., exercise, purging).

*Possible direction:* Details on exactly what your client is consuming will be very valuable in this scenario—we do not want to make assumptions. In this case, collecting specific food data will help to guide you and your client. Writing "sandwich with milk and cookies" at lunch does not provide enough information to determine what exactly is being consumed. Instead, coach your client to be behaviorally specific (e.g., two slices of white bread with 1 tbsp of mayo, 1 tbsp of butter, two pieces of chicken breast, lettuce, 1 slice of cheddar cheese, 1 cup of 2% milk, two chocolate chip cookies from Starbucks).

*Scenario 2:* Your client has low potassium due to purging and laxative use (T1). They demonstrate a pattern of obsessionality and perfectionism that has gotten in the way with accurate tracking (T2).

*Possible direction:* The goal at this time is getting out of medical instability. The most effective solution may be to have the client provide some detail about food intake without the minutia at this time. Instead, the focus is on tracking purging and laxative use as this leads to unstable electrolytes. That said, sometimes more detail is necessary to find the missing links (e.g., client engages in purging when they consume butter or oils; a detail you might not have if you keep the tracking more general).

It is important to remember that your client will likely vacillate between needing a lot of detail and not needing too much detail. We appreciate that this might make you feel uncertain or want more concrete steps or directions. This is where we rely on dialectical theory, DBT assumptions about therapy, and consultation team meetings to ensure that we are following the model, staying effective (rather than "right"), and not engaging in therapy-interfering behaviors.

As you can see, part of being effective in this model rests on your (and your team's) knowledge of eating and meal planning. Knowing when to increase or decrease meal planning, helping your client develop skills to create grocery lists, and correctly interpreting whether there is "enough" intake is very difficult without proper training in nutrition sciences. As a result, and based on your training background, some of you will feel more comfortable with this than others. If you do not feel you have the necessary skill set, relying on a dietitian will be important.

## Hunger and Fullness Scale

As we know, many clients with eating disorders do not have accurate or particularly strong, hunger and fullness cues. Although some clients may never develop reliable interoceptive abilities, we felt it was important to encourage some appetite awareness training on the diary card. As such, we ask clients to rate any observable sensations of hunger and fullness at the start and at the end of each meal. While some clients can do this relatively easily, it can take months for some clients to notice and rate these cues, while others may never have definitive hunger and fullness cues. Tracking these cues can help clients increase mindful awareness of "empty" and "full" sensations and begin to put words around their experience.

Tracking hunger and fullness cues can also provide relevant data to explain why eating might be challenging. For example, we have had clients note very high fullness cues first thing in the morning, despite not having eaten since their evening snack. Given recent findings showing that some individuals with ARFID produce elevated levels of cholecystokinin (a hormone that signals fullness) in the mornings, we wonder if a possible phenomenon is happening transdiagnostically and impacting willingness or desire to eat. This type of information can alter the treatment approach (e.g., addressing lack of appetite is different from targeting a fear of eating a particular food). Regardless of your client's degree of interoceptive awareness, it is helpful to help them build skills that facilitate eating in the context of unstable hunger and satiety cues.

## Location

Your client can also track *where* they ate/drank. This aids in determining helpful or unhelpful patterns with respect to feeding routines and rituals. For example, some clients may report eating frequently in their car, while working at their desk, or only when standing. This type of information can help when trying to normalize food routines or interrupt patterns that contribute to targeted behaviors.

## Fluid Intake

Your client uses this column to track the amount and type of fluid consumed each day. This helps you and your client determine the risk of medical instability (e.g., in the case of excessive water intake or severe dehydration) as well as potential functional relationships between fluid intake/fluid restriction and coping with emotions or physical distress (e.g., excessive consumption of water or ice in an effort to thwart hunger cues).

## Symptom Columns

The next eight columns are meant to be customized to your client treatment plan and include spaces to track both ED behaviors and traditional DBT targets (e.g., suicide attempts, self-injury, substance use). Our template includes common targets in MED-DBT, and you can change those or use the blank column spaces for other relevant targets. Even when symptoms subside it is important to keep tracking urges over the course of treatment as they commonly wax and wane. When reporting on an urge or symptom, your client will either place an "X" in the box if they engaged in the behavior, or rate the urge from "0" (no urge) to "5" (most intense urge imaginable). We ask our clients to fill in each box and not to leave them blank. This allows you to quickly scan each diary card, taking note of high urges and "X's" to set the agenda for the session.

## Emotions Today and Ratings

Given the centrality of emotion regulation in this model, your client will reflect each day on their affective experience and rate their emotions using a Likert scale, where "0" means "I did not feel this emotion today" to "5" for "I felt the most intense expression of this emotion today." We ask clients to rate the highest intensity for the day, even if the duration was brief. For example, it is important to know that a client reaches a "5" every day in disgust, even just briefly. Keep in mind that many of our clients are not familiar with or comfortable sharing information about emotions. Explain that the emotion names listed on the diary card are meant to capture all iterations of that particular feeling. In other words, when reflecting on whether your client felt anxious, they would consider edginess, apprehension, horror, nervousness, worry, and overwhelm under that category. Clients also sometimes deny experiencing anger; however, when that is expanded to include rage, hostility, bitterness, frustration, or aggravation, they do recognize those experiences under this category. In this way, the diary card becomes another helpful way of teaching emotional literacy and identification.

## Urge to Quit Treatment or Recovery

Ambivalence about treatment and recovery, lack of insight into the seriousness of the ED, and the ego-syntonic nature of many ED behaviors are par for the course. Motivation waxes and wanes; therefore, having a place to capture fluctuating thoughts and feelings about staying in treatment helps to keep them front and center for you and your client. We ask clients to rate their urges from "0" for "I don't have any urges to quit" to "5" for "extremely high urges to quit treatment or recovery."

## Keeping Secrets

Withholding information in treatment makes it difficult to accurately understand our clients and help them build lives worth living. We do not judge clients for keeping secrets because we know they serve a function. Instead, we ask clients to be mindful of the secrets they keep and to rate the urge to do so in treatment from 0 to 5 or to mark an "X" if they are, in fact, already withholding information. Let your client know that the expectation is not that they *must* disclose what they are withholding; rather, the aim is to be aware that there are secrets, to explore the pros and cons of not being forthcoming, and to not avoid the fact that it is happening. Ironically, we find that our clients tend to tell us what the secret is simply because we don't demand to know it!

## PART B: Tracking Skills

Diary cards also serve the important function of tracking skill use and reminding clients that there are many skill options to choose from when managing difficult situations. Using the weekly chart provided on the diary card, your client will circle the skill used by day. This helps you and your client evaluate whether skills are being used and if there are patterns to the skills used versus not used.

### Identify and Troubleshoot What Might Get in the Way of Using Diary Cards

MED-DBT diary cards are an exposure exercise and can feel overwhelming for clients and practitioners. For this reason, it is important to observe, identify, and discuss potential obstacles that you or your client might face in tracking these behaviors. This conversation starts during pretreatment but will come up in various ways over the course of therapy. Some clients do not want to think about what they have eaten, while others rigidly count calories and ruminate about meal prep, food processing, and menu planning. Clinicians have reported to us that it can be tempting to stop tracking altogether or to become so hyper-focused on the intake themselves that they cannot "see the forest for the trees." For these reasons, it is crucial that you are mindful of common obstacles and feel prepared to manage ambivalence in you and your client when it inevitably shows up.

In this section, we share some common thoughts, emotions, and behaviors that get in the way of completing diary cards. For each obstacle listed below, we recommend that you maintain a dialectical stance, modeling acceptance of your client's position and validating the wisdom in their perspective while simultaneously pushing for change. Always keep in mind the nutritional status of your client. EDs by nature cause widespread dysregulation cognitively, emotionally, and behaviorally. The ability of your client to remember information and stay regulated can be greatly impacted by malnourishment and other ED behaviors (e.g., exhaustion due to excessive exercise). Patience, compassion, and a dialectical worldview are of utmost importance.

*Obstacle #1:* Your client reports that tracking food/fluid makes their ED worse because it is "just like counting calories/dieting."

*Recommended approach:* Validate that this really hard exercise can (on first glance) remind them of calorie counting or past dieting approaches. Assess what specific elements about the tracking are making their ED worse. For example, is it reporting on food in general? Having to look at a binge episode in detail? Observing hunger and fullness cues? Remain both curious and dialectical and validate the truth in their perspective. Reorient to the rationale for tracking food and fluid intake. Unlike dieting methods or the ED itself, we are not counting calories, labeling food as good or bad, or tracking for the purposes of weight loss. Use a foot-in-the-door/door-in-the-face sequence to increase commitment to trying the diary card (e.g., "What would it be like to fill it out for a few days this week and talk about your experience at our next session?").

For some clients, taking pictures of their meals and snacks can be a way to track more easily. This may be helpful for those with learning or visual-spatial differences that make writing or using the existing diary card layout difficult. You will want to assess whether photographing food serves an avoidant function for your client. We have been told that writing down food intake is more direct and emotionally challenging than taking a picture. We have also observed that viewing numerous photos of food in addition to reviewing the rest of the diary card can be cumbersome for clinicians. The goal is to find an effective solution to collecting the data. If you are getting lost in the data, this is not effective! Your client may also benefit from using different apps to track urges and behaviors. At the time of this writing, available apps do not include all of the functions of the MED-DBT diary card; therefore, you will need to work with your client to determine whether a particular app will be useful.

Finally, remind your client that MED-DBT is an emotion-based model, which means that we don't want to avoid our feelings. Getting triggered and feeling uncomfortable will be a natural part of the recovery process and the treatment is designed to help your client navigate that in a way that doesn't feel insurmountable.

*Obstacle #2:* Your client tells you that tracking binge-eating episodes causes too much shame and shouldn't be something they write down.

*Recommended approach:* Unlike some ED symptoms that are ego-syntonic—meaning they align with the client's sense of self and are not experienced as problematic—other symptoms like binge eating are typically accompanied by varying degrees of shame. Binge episodes are typically done in secret to ensure privacy and to lessen intense emotion. Most clients do not want to talk about or write down the details of a binge. Providing psychoeducation about EDs, how shame shows up in EDs, and linking back to the adapted biosocial theory is a helpful way to validate your client's experiences and needs. It makes sense that tracking a binge episode would be difficult. When this happens, you might explore when and how your client has been invalidated for overeating or binge eating in the past. How has diet culture played a role? What type of communications occurred in their family or peer groups that would contribute to a feeling of shame around binge eating? Are there cultural components at play here that we are missing?

This is also an area where reminding clients about the genetic and neurobiological underpinnings of binge eating is key. The shame may be part of a belief that they "should" have more self-control and that they "should" be able to override the urge to binge. Highlighting that binge eating is not a willpower or self-control problem, it is a biosocial problem that requires specialized treatment. Using your levels of validation (Linehan, 1997), talk with your client about why it is so important to know when they binge, as well as where and with what food. Knowing how often binge episodes occur helps us refine meal planning and skill use. Understanding patterns with respect to the time of day allows us to uncover physiological and psychological factors driving the behavior. Learning about the types of foods eaten during the day versus during a binge helps to determine potential nutritional deficits that further drive cravings and urges. Your job is to use a matter-of-fact and nonjudgmental manner when discussing these topics with your clients. It is important to both validate the valid and help clients check the facts, or act opposite to shame when it makes sense to do so rather than avoid tracking symptoms.

*Obstacle #3:* Your client is tracking food in a very general manner when you need more specific details.

*Recommended approach:* Often, and more so in the early stages of treatment, you may receive diary cards that are only partially completed or that lack detail with respect to food and fluid quantity. Shape effective behavior by reinforcing that they brought the diary card to the session and attempted to fill it in. Without judgment, observe that some details are missing. It is important not to make assumptions about why the food section was completed in this manner. Instead, use a missing links analysis to explore the factors that contributed to the behavior. Did your client understand what was expected? Did they remember the instructions? Were they willing to do it? Do they have the skills to track food and fluid intake in detail? Does not writing down food in detail serve a protective or regulating function? Could this be a way of avoiding talking about eating or something else? The answers to these questions will guide your intervention.

In general, discuss with your client why you both agreed to track food intake in this manner and how it links to the target hierarchy and, importantly, to *their* LWL goals. Reorient to the rationale that knowing specific quantities helps you both be more efficient with meal planning, mitigating medical risks, and identifying patterns of unbalanced intake. Ultimately, this will help your client learn to feed themselves in a manner that, at minimum, keeps them alive and, maximally, contributes to sustaining their LWL goals.

*Obstacle #4:* Your client says that tracking symptoms in this manner reinforces perfectionism/rigidity.

*Recommended approach:* While it is often the case that individuals with EDs struggle with overcontrolled characteristics, learning to engage with food, eating, and body image are core skills in MED-DBT. Certainly, some clients will approach food in a highly ritualized, ruminative, and compulsive manner. Avoiding the diary card for this reason serves to reinforce the notion that they are unable to find a dialectical way of relating to food or managing emotions. This can be a useful time to explain or reorient to the dialectical tension between having no meal plan/not tracking at all versus rigidly and minutely tracking food (see Chapter 7 on dialectical dilemmas): neither extreme is beneficial for our clients. The goal is to find a middle path with respect to feeding and physical health. Thus, it is necessary at this stage of treatment for your client to know what they are eating, when, and how.

Rather than removing food tracking as a way to manage inflexibility, clinicians lean into dialectics and introduce other ways to engage with the diary card that are more spontaneous, flexible, and even playful. We remind clients that MED-DBT is designed to help people move away from extreme ways of thinking, feeling, and acting. This is true for those with over- and undercontrolled coping styles. Over time, those who tend to avoid food and eating learn to approach it while those who engage from a place of perfectionism and rigid control learn to nourish themselves with greater flexibility. Both coping styles need help interacting with food!

*Obstacle #5:* You avoid the food portion of the diary card due to your own discomfort with targeting nutrition.

*Recommended approach:* When we engage in TIBs, we make lemonade out of those lemons and use that as an opportunity to both out ourselves to our clients (e.g., fallibility agreement) and consult with them about how to do better. It may be that your client can help you head off your avoidance by contributing to a more thorough review of eating in session. It might mean that increased support from an ED-trained dietitian is needed. It may also mean that you need to spend more time learning about food and fluid intake from an ED lens or work on what might be getting in the way with your consult team or an outside consultant.

### Use Contingency Management Strategies to Shape Effective Behavior

Incomplete diary cards are therapy-interfering and are targeted as such in individual sessions. Contingency management protocols refer to collaborative and strategically placed consequences that you and your client agree to observe when a target behavior occurs. Contingencies are not to be used in a punishing or pejorative manner, and it is important that clients understand the definition and rationale for the use of these procedures. Ideas for shaping an incomplete diary card might include the following:

- Using a missing links or chain analysis to understand the factors that control or maintain the behavior
- Using session time to discuss what got in the way
- Discussing pros and cons of completing diary card
- Increasing use of DBT commitment strategies (e.g., devil's advocate, freedom to choose)

If you and your client agree on what is getting in the way, and the above interventions did not shape the behavior, you can introduce stronger consequences (ideally with your client's collaboration). These might include the following:

- Asking your client to return to the waiting room to complete their diary cards without extending session time
- Withdrawing warmth when your client hands in another incomplete diary card
- Requesting diary cards to be sent in via email 1 hour before your scheduled session in order to meet with you

Once the behavior resolves, the contingency is removed, thus rewarding your client for the effective action. Diary cards are hard work; therefore, it is important for you to use reinforcement strategies to encourage effective behavior. Examples of reinforcement include acknowledging your client's willingness to track food and fluid intake when it is aversive to them, smiling and using an easy manner when completed diary cards are provided, removing the need to discuss ambivalence about diary cards during sessions when they are done, and expressing excitement or appreciation when the appetite awareness continuum is used.

## Summary

Diary cards are central to MED-DBT. The adaptations to the original DBT diary cards ensure that both ED behaviors are tracked alongside suicide, self-injury, and other emotion regulation difficulties. While they can be a steep learning curve for you and your client, they provide great therapeutic value. Hang in there! Introduce them early in treatment and give your client a few weeks to get used to them. Plan to spend time in session reviewing them and ensuring that they are being completed fully and accurately. When met with ambivalence, validate, stay dialectical, assess the variables getting in the way, and work collaboratively with your client to move forward. Once diary cards are in place and clients are tracking key behaviors, urges, and emotions, the next step is to use that information to drive insight and change. In the following chapter, we explore how to apply two of DBT's most effective change-based tools—behavior-chain analysis and missing links analysis—to help clients understand the function of their behaviors and identify new, more skillful ways to respond.

**Handout 13.1**

**MED-DBT DIARY CARD: PART A**

| Time of Day | MEALS | Food Intake—Include approximate quantity and description of food<br>Hunger Scale—Graph hunger level from start to end of meal | Location | Fluid Intake | Suicide | NSSI | Restrict | Binge | Purge | Exercise | | | Emotions Today | Rating (0-5) |
|---|---|---|---|---|---|---|---|---|---|---|---|---|---|---|
| | Name: | Day/Date: | | | Mark (*) if you engaged in behavior. Rate (0–5) if you had an urge but did not engage in behavior. | | | | | | | | | |
| | **BREAKFAST** | empty \| 2 \| 3 \| 4 \| neutral \| 6 \| 7 \| 8 \| 9 \| full | | | | | | | | | | | Anxiety<br>Happy<br>Sad | _____<br>_____<br>_____ |
| | **SNACK** | empty \| 2 \| 3 \| 4 \| neutral \| 6 \| 7 \| 8 \| 9 \| full | | | | | | | | | | | Shame<br>Anger | _____<br>_____ |
| | **LUNCH** | empty \| 2 \| 3 \| 4 \| neutral \| 6 \| 7 \| 8 \| 9 \| full | | | | | | | | | | | Guilt<br>Disgust<br>Envy | _____<br>_____<br>_____ |
| | **SNACK** | empty \| 2 \| 3 \| 4 \| neutral \| 6 \| 7 \| 8 \| 9 \| full | | | | | | | | | | | Urge to quit Tx/ recovery | _____ |
| | **DINNER** | empty \| 2 \| 3 \| 4 \| neutral \| 6 \| 7 \| 8 \| 9 \| full | | | | | | | | | | | Urge to keep secrets<br>Urge to lie | _____<br>_____ |
| | **SNACK** | empty \| 2 \| 3 \| 4 \| neutral \| 6 \| 7 \| 8 \| 9 \| full | | | | | | | | | | | | |

Copyright © 2026 Anita Federici and Lucene Wisniewski. From *Treating Eating Disorders with DBT* by Anita Federici and Lucene Wisniewski, published by The Guilford Press (2026). Permission to photocopy this material, or to download and print enlarged versions (*www.guilford.com/federici-forms*), is granted to purchasers of this book for personal use only; see copyright page for details.

Handout 13.1 (*continued*)

**MED-DBT DIARY CARD: PART B**

| **What skills did I try/practice/use this week to get through? Circle the days you worked on each skill.** | | | | | | | |
|---|---|---|---|---|---|---|---|
| 1. Activating Wise Mind | Monday | Tuesday | Wednesday | Thursday | Friday | Saturday | Sunday |
| 2. Observe: Just Notice (Urge Surfing) | Monday | Tuesday | Wednesday | Thursday | Friday | Saturday | Sunday |
| 3. Describe: Put Words On | Monday | Tuesday | Wednesday | Thursday | Friday | Saturday | Sunday |
| 4. Participate: Enter into the Experience | Monday | Tuesday | Wednesday | Thursday | Friday | Saturday | Sunday |
| 5. Nonjudgmental Stance | Monday | Tuesday | Wednesday | Thursday | Friday | Saturday | Sunday |
| 6. One-Mindfully: Doing One Thing at a Time | Monday | Tuesday | Wednesday | Thursday | Friday | Saturday | Sunday |
| 7. Effectiveness: Focus on What Works | Monday | Tuesday | Wednesday | Thursday | Friday | Saturday | Sunday |
| 8. Wise Mind **ACCEPTS** | Monday | Tuesday | Wednesday | Thursday | Friday | Saturday | Sunday |
| 9. Self-Soothe with five senses | Monday | Tuesday | Wednesday | Thursday | Friday | Saturday | Sunday |
| 10. STOP skill | Monday | Tuesday | Wednesday | Thursday | Friday | Saturday | Sunday |
| 11. **IMPROVE** the Moment | Monday | Tuesday | Wednesday | Thursday | Friday | Saturday | Sunday |
| 12. **TIPP (when medically stable)** | Monday | Tuesday | Wednesday | Thursday | Friday | Saturday | Sunday |
| 13. Pros and Cons | Monday | Tuesday | Wednesday | Thursday | Friday | Saturday | Sunday |
| 14. Radical Acceptance | Monday | Tuesday | Wednesday | Thursday | Friday | Saturday | Sunday |
| 15. Reduce Vulnerability: **PLEASE** | Monday | Tuesday | Wednesday | Thursday | Friday | Saturday | Sunday |
| 16. Accumulate Positives | Monday | Tuesday | Wednesday | Thursday | Friday | Saturday | Sunday |
| 17. Build **MASTERY** | Monday | Tuesday | Wednesday | Thursday | Friday | Saturday | Sunday |
| 18. Cope Ahead | Monday | Tuesday | Wednesday | Thursday | Friday | Saturday | Sunday |
| 19. Check the Facts | Monday | Tuesday | Wednesday | Thursday | Friday | Saturday | Sunday |
| 20. Opposite-to-Emotion Action | Monday | Tuesday | Wednesday | Thursday | Friday | Saturday | Sunday |
| 21. Acted on my Values/Life Worth Living Goals | Monday | Tuesday | Wednesday | Thursday | Friday | Saturday | Sunday |
| 22. Problem Solving | Monday | Tuesday | Wednesday | Thursday | Friday | Saturday | Sunday |
| 23. Dialectical Thinking | Monday | Tuesday | Wednesday | Thursday | Friday | Saturday | Sunday |
| 24. Used Positive Reinforcement or Contingencies | Monday | Tuesday | Wednesday | Thursday | Friday | Saturday | Sunday |
| 25. Objective Effectiveness: **DEAR MAN** | Monday | Tuesday | Wednesday | Thursday | Friday | Saturday | Sunday |
| 26. Relationship Effectiveness: **GIVE** | Monday | Tuesday | Wednesday | Thursday | Friday | Saturday | Sunday |
| 27. Self-Respect Effectiveness: **FAST** | Monday | Tuesday | Wednesday | Thursday | Friday | Saturday | Sunday |

## Handout 13.2

### How to Use MED-DBT Diary Cards

Diary cards are an important part of your treatment plan. This handout explains why we use diary cards and provides step-by-step instructions on how to fill them out.

### Why Use Diary Cards?

- Diary cards are **the fastest way to communicate large amounts of information** about yourself to your therapist. When there is so much going on, it would take most of the session just to get caught up on the details of the week, leaving little time to effectively work on feeling better. By completing diary cards, you ensure that your therapist has the best possible chance of getting to know you and understanding what your week was like, as quickly as possible.
- Diary cards are used to **set the agenda** for your therapy sessions so that high-priority items (e.g., behaviors that could result in death or interfere with treatment) don't get left to the last minute. Together with your therapist, you will use the information on your diary card to structure your therapy hour efficiently, which will help you reach your life worth living goals more effectively.
- **Aids in accurate recall**. It is very difficult to remember what one ate last week, how intense an urge was 5 days ago, or what one's hunger and fullness cues were in retrospect. In order to understand your unique experiences, your therapist needs the most accurate data from you! This is also an important way to reduce misunderstandings.
- Allows you to **identify important patterns and relationships** between ED urges/behaviors and your emotions or other behaviors (e.g., self-injury, substance use). It can be hard to make sense of our experiences without tracking how they arise and what factors contribute to them.
- **Increases awareness and reduces avoidance** of eating habits and ED symptoms. Diary cards are a very mindful activity and they help us observe and describe the things we might tend to avoid.

Copyright © 2026 Anita Federici and Lucene Wisniewski. From *Treating Eating Disorders with DBT* by Anita Federici and Lucene Wisniewski, published by The Guilford Press (2026). Permission to photocopy this material, or to download and print enlarged versions (*www.guilford.com/federici-forms*), is granted to purchasers of this book for personal use only; see copyright page for details.

## How to Fill Out the Diary Card?

Your MED-DBT diary card has two parts:

**Part A** tracks food and fluid intake; eating disorder symptoms, suicidal and self-injurious urges, behaviors, and emotions; and other behaviors that you are struggling with.

**Part B** helps you track the skills you use.
Diary cards are to be completed *each day*. It can be helpful to schedule the same time each day to complete your diary card and to use a reminder so you don't forget. Choose a place where you have privacy to fill them out and find a safe place to store them.

### PART A

**Time of Day:** It is important to track *when* you eat and drink. This helps us identify restrictive or delayed patterns of eating or other trends with respect to your relationship with food. Try to be as accurate as possible when entering the time of day. This column can also be used to facilitate mechanical eating by pre-populating the times that you plan to eat meals and snacks.

**Food Intake:** Use this section to write down what was eaten, including a description of the food and the quantity. This level of detail provides important data about your relationship with food and how you approach eating. Writing "*ate a sandwich with milk and cookies*" at lunch does not provide enough information. Instead, please provide more detail (e.g., two slices of white bread with 1 tbsp of mayo, 1 tbsp of butter, two pieces of chicken breast, lettuce, 1 slice of cheddar cheese, 1 cup of 2% milk, two chocolate chip cookies). If you are working with a dietitian, they can also review this section with you.

**Hunger Scale:** Many people with eating disorders do not have accurate or available hunger and fullness cues. As part of appetite awareness training, we ask you to try and rate your hunger and fullness at the start of each meal and then again at the end of the meal. We know that many people struggle with this activity and it may take several months before hunger and fullness cues begin to stabilize. It may also be the case that these interoceptive cues are always unreliable, in which case diary cards can help you learn to eat even when you are unsure of hunger and fullness.

**Location:** Enter *where* you ate/drank each meal and snack. This helps to determine helpful or unhelpful patterns with respect to feeding routines and rituals. For example, you may observe that you frequently eat in your car or while working at your desk. Helping you to evaluate styles and patterns of eating are an important part of treatment.

**Fluid Intake:** Similar to the food intake column, tracking the amount and type of fluid consumed each day is very helpful. If the time of fluid intake differs from the "Time of Day" column in which you ate a meal, please note that on your diary card. This section is used to track all fluid intake, including water, coffee, diet and regular products, and alcohol.

**Symptom Columns:** In the MED-DBT program it is essential to include all relevant ED behaviors (e.g., binge eating, purging, restricting, exercise, chewing/spitting, etc.) alongside behaviors related to emotion dysregulation (e.g., suicide, self-injury, substance use, dissociation). You will work with your therapist to customize this section to your specific needs and treatment goals. Even when symptoms subside it is important to keep tracking them over the course of treatment as they commonly wax and wane. Please track symptoms as follows:

- Place an "X" in the box if you engaged in the behavior,

  OR

- If you had an urge *but did not engage* in the behavior, rate the urge from "0" for "no urge" *to* "5" for "most intense urge imaginable."

**Emotions Today and Ratings:** Take time each day to reflect on your emotions. Rate each one on a scale from "0" for "I did not feel this emotion today" to "5" for "I experienced the most intense expression of this emotion today." Your therapist will help you understand your different emotions so you can accurately identify what you are feeling. Rate the highest number for the day, even if the intensity of the emotion was brief. For example, it is important to know that you experienced a "5" every day with anger, even if it was for a few short moments. Talk to your therapist about what the ratings mean so you are on the same page. It is helpful to note that the emotion name listed on the diary card represents a range of experiences. For instance, *anxiety* captures edginess, apprehension, horror, nervousness, worry, and overwhelm. *Anger* captures rage, hostility, bitterness, frustration, aggravation.

**Urge to Quit Treatment or Recovery:** Ambivalence and commitment to treatment wax and wane over time. This is normal! Having a place to capture fluctuating feelings helps us keep them front and center so we can explore them in therapy. Please rate your urges from "0" for "I don't have any urges to quit" to "5" for "extremely high urges to quit treatment or recovery."

### Lying and Withholding

**Urges to Lie:** Lying is adding or changing information in a way that creates a false understanding. It's when someone misrepresents the truth or provides information that is not true. This is different from withholding information.

**Urges to Keep Secrets:** Keeping a secret or withholding information is choosing not to share something—it's about what is left out rather than what is said. Sometimes, this is to protect privacy, avoid conflict, or because you may not be ready to share.

Use the diary card to track urges or behaviors related to lying or withholding (i.e., keeping secrets). This gives us an opportunity to observe the behavior and explore what the function of it might be. While you do not have to tell your therapist *what* you are withholding or lying about, we ask you to rate either the urge to withhold information and/or to lie (on a scale of 0–5) or identify that you are actively holding back information and/or lying by placing an "X" in the appropriate space.

**Both lying and withholding can shape how others perceive a situation, but the key difference is whether new, inaccurate information is introduced (lying) or if certain details are simply not shared (omission).**

### PART B

Throughout the week, please track which DBT and ED recovery skills you used by circling the day a particular skill was used. While not an exhaustive list, the selected skills on the diary card help remind you about other ways to cope and to evaluate (1) whether skills are being used and (2) whether there are patterns of skills used versus not used.

### What if I have difficulty filling out my diary cards?

Diary cards can be overwhelming and they take time to get used to. This is normal! Please talk to your therapist about what is getting in the way so they can help you.

# 14

# Behavior-Chain Analysis and Missing Links Analysis in MED-DBT

You and your client are targeting medical instability caused by recurrent daily episodes of purging. He is followed by a doctor who has recommended the use of potassium supplements and seeking emergency room care when he feels unwell, including chest pains or dizziness. While he agrees in session to follow these recommendations, he struggles to do them in the moment. He has gone to the ER twice in 48 hours and was admitted for intravenous fluids the second time. Upon returning home from the ER, he engaged in several episodes of binge eating and purging requiring yet another ER visit. As his therapist, you are feeling at a loss. There seems to be agreement in session to focus on life-threatening behavior but this appears to unravel between sessions. Why does this keep happening in spite of your efforts and his stated willingness? Why does the behavior persist even though it is ruining your client's life? You are starting to have thoughts that maybe he doesn't really want to get better.

Comfortably positioned alongside acceptance-based strategies, DBT employs a number of change-based interventions in an effort to move a client closer to their life worth living goals. Central to DBT's extensive package of problem-solving strategies are two powerhouse interventions: behavior-chain analysis and missing links analysis. Both are designed to increase awareness about problem behaviors and to empower your client to begin to see that they have many more options to manage than they imagined. Together you learn that their actions make sense and they can create change if they want to.

## What Are Behavior-Chain Analysis and Missing Links Analysis?

Behavior-chain analysis (BCA) plays a central role in MED-DBT. Highly detailed in nature, BCA captures a snapshot in time and provides detail on the variables that shape and control the target behavior. It is designed to help you and your client develop a much more nuanced and thorough understanding of why a behavior happens again and again, despite numerous efforts to modify or change it. While BCA is primarily applied to behaviors that have happened (e.g., purging, exercise, laxative use, self-injury), a missing links analysis (MLA) targets the absence of behavior (e.g., food restriction, missed medical appointments). As two primary change-based strategies, it is essential that clinicians utilizing MED-DBT feel confident orienting clients to and delivering adherent BCAs and MLAs. For a detailed description of these interventions, we recommend Shireen Rizvi's (2019) book on the subject.

While our standard DBT colleagues will be familiar with these interventions, there are important nuances and differences when applied to ED behaviors that we detail in this chapter. For those trained in standard ED protocols, BCA and MLA protocols are likely new interventions and may require more training and consultation. Practice both BCA and MLA protocols on yourself and with colleagues to increase your ease and familiarity with them. Make sure that you feel comfortable using these interventions before teaching them to your client. Then orient/reorient your client to the purpose and rationale of using BCAs/MLAs. While you will have covered this in the pretreatment phase, your clients will benefit from commitment strategies and micro-orienting to the rationale as needed over time.

Chain analysis is an in-depth process that rests on collaboration and a trusting therapeutic relationship. BCAs and MLAs are designed to be practiced with willingness, curiosity, and a shared agreement to explore target behaviors without judgment. While these interventions will occur as the result of a behavior (e.g., an MLA for a missed dinner), it can be a fine line between exploring to understand versus using a chain analysis to punish a client for engaging in a behavior. It is important not to drag your clients through a chain, *and* sometimes it is necessary. If a BCA or an MLA is needed, observe and describe the need with your client. For example:

"I can understand your request not to do a chain today because you are feeling really tired. I am also noticing my wise mind reminding me about an earlier conversation about the role of avoidance in your life. I am going to ask us to work through the chain even though you feel tired and maybe we can use some self-soothing skills along the way to make it feel less taxing?"

One of the reasons we ask clinicians to do their own chain analyses is because there is tremendous value in experiencing the vulnerability required to complete the process. We find that clinicians who have worked through their own BCAs and MLAs are more likely to use them and are able to stay dialectical through the process (offering timely validation while pushing for change). These change-based strategies apply "heat" to vulnerable behaviors. Like all exposure strategies, we are asking clients to face commonly avoided feelings and thoughts, and to talk openly about behaviors that often elicit anxiety, shame, and guilt (e.g., binge eating, chewing and spitting). Talk with your clients about the process, share your own experience doing a BCA, and develop a cope ahead plan (e.g., holding ice, using a weighted blanket) to maximize success.

## How BCAs and MLAs Help Clients with EDs

It may seem counterintuitive to ask a client to track emotions, urges, and actions when they struggle with decreased insight or anosognosia (a brain-based condition that interferes with a person's ability to accurately perceive the seriousness of their illness). In our experience, the use of BCAs and MLAs can be incredibly helpful in building awareness and decreasing confusion. For example, one client initially reported that she binged "out of nowhere" and felt like she had no control or warning signs. However, through several BCAs, she began to notice that her binge episodes were consistently preceded by long periods of restrictive eating, high interpersonal stress, and intense self-critical thoughts. Over time, she was able to recognize these patterns earlier and begin using alternative skills, ultimately reducing her binge frequency and feeling more in control.

Many of our clients have long histories of being misunderstood or told they are "too complex" or not in a "recovery mindset." It is not uncommon for others to make assumptions about why a person isn't eating or engaging in ED or self-injurious behavior (e.g., they just want to lose weight, they just want to get my attention). But behaviors serve powerful functions and it is important that we do not impose our assumptions or biases onto our clients. The things that prompt and maintain your client's symptoms are probably not the things most people think about, otherwise other treatment approaches would have solved the problem by now. It is more likely the case that the factors reinforcing your client's symptoms are less obvious and more intricate or layered. Change cannot occur if we have a limited understanding of why a behavior keeps happening, so we use BCAs and MLAs to be much more precise.

On a related note, by the time they get to you, your client may be feeling quite hopeless about their future. A client reported to us that they were told years ago that they would always have an eating disorder and would likely die young. We do not believe this to be true for our clients. BCAs and MLAs create openings by allowing our clients to begin to understand their own behaviors. At the very least, they shine a light on all the different ways the chain could work out differently and lead to different outcomes. BCAs and MLAs are emotion-focused and guided by ED biotemperament. Exploring causes and maintaining factors is not unique to adult ED treatment. CBT-E utilizes a binge-analysis worksheet, exposure hierarchies, and thought records to better understand behavioral patterns and to elicit exposure to beliefs and assumptions that influence actions. However, BCAs are much more detailed with respect to observing emotional shifts and bodily sensations unique to EDs that are incredibly helpful for our clients. The moment-by-moment analysis of a BCA better captures the interplay of emotion, cognition, urges, actions, and physical changes that led to and maintain behaviors.

## MLA Example for Food Restriction

Let's use the case study from the start of this chapter. Your client had recommendations from their doctor to use potassium supplements to counter the effects of purging on his heart and to go to the ER when feeling unwell. While he was reporting to the ER, he was not taking the prescribed potassium supplements. An MLA can help you determine why the behavior is not happening.

*Therapist*: Okay, let's use our missing links analysis questions to figure out what might be happening with the potassium supplements.

*Client*: Sure.

*Therapist*: What is the first question on the MLA?

*Client*: (*looking at his handout*) Well, it says, "did I know what effective behavior was needed or expected?"

*Therapist*: What was your experience? Did you know that you were supposed to take the supplements?

### Scenario 1: Client Was Not Clear on What to Do

*Client: I knew I should take them, but I wasn't sure when. Like, every day? Or only when I purge? And like, what if I purge, take a supplement and then purge again? Should I take another one?*

*Therapist*: Those are really great questions. What do you think got in the way of knowing what you needed to do?

*Client*: Probably because I hate going to talk to my doctor so I tuned out our conversation.

*Therapist*: Yeah, that'll do it! So how do we solve this problem?

*Client*: Probably listen better!

*Therapist*: LOL, not sure that really addresses how nervous you feel talking to your doctor!

*Client*: No, I guess not. I would need to be more grounded, or maybe bring my friend with me. Maybe I could record the session or take notes or something.

*Therapist*: Those are all great ideas. Let's work on those, but we also need to figure out how your doctor wants you to use those supplements.

*Client*: I guess I could call the office?

*Therapist*: That's a good idea. Why don't you do that now?

### Scenario 2: Client Was Clear on What to Do and Was Not Willing to Do It

*Therapist: What was your experience? Did you know that you were supposed to take the supplements?*

*Client*: Yeah, I've had to use them before so I know what to do.

*Therapist*: Okay, what's the next MLA question?

*Client*: Was I willing to do what was needed? (*Pauses.*) Yeah, that's a solid no.

*Therapist*: Well! I appreciate the directness. What got in the way of wanting to do what was needed or planned?

*Client*: I don't think I need them. Really, it's overkill.

*Therapist*: Ah, okay so you know what to do but don't agree that they are needed? Is that right?

*Client*: Like, I get that I might need them sometimes. I don't want to have heart problems but when I am at home and I've just purged, I actually feel fine, sometimes I even feel better so I don't feel the need to supplement.

*Therapist*: I appreciate the clarification because you and I have talked about why you would use these supplements. So, the willingness is there under certain circumstances but not all instances of purging?

*Client*: Yeah and like, sometimes I get really bad stomachaches when I take those supplements so I don't want to take them unless I really need them.

*Therapist*: Yeah, that is a lousy side effect. It sounds like we need to get clarification from your doctor about your questions and about managing the side effects. Are you willing to do that?

*Client*: Yeah, I can do that. I wouldn't mind asking her if there is another option.

### Scenario 3: Client Was Clear on What to Do and Was Willing to Do It, but Didn't Think about It

*Therapist: What was your experience? Did you know that you were supposed to take the supplements?*

*Client*: Yeah, I've had to use them before so I know what to do.

*Therapist*: Okay, what's the next MLA question?

*Client*: Was I willing to do what was needed? (*Pauses.*) Yeah! I was.

*Therapist*: Okay, what comes next on the MLA worksheet?

*Client*: Did the thought of doing what was needed or expected ever enter my mind? (*Pauses to think.*) It didn't! I was so exhausted after that last binge-purge episode that I got into bed and passed out!

*Therapist*: The exhaustion is understandable. Those cycles of binge eating and purging are very hard on the mind and body. I appreciate that you were willing to use the supplements. What do you think we could do differently to remind you to take them under similar circumstances?

*Client*: Oh, geez! I would have to literally trip over them to remember when I'm in that state.

*Therapist*: Actually, that's not a bad idea. How could you make it so you literally trip over them?

*Client*: Uh, maybe leave the bottle on my pillow? Or put a big note on my dresser so I see it every day? I guess I could set an alarm reminder too because the symptoms are happening around the same time at night.

*Therapist*: Love those ideas. Can we implement them today?

### Scenario 4: Client Was Clear on What to Do and Was Willing to Do It, Thought about It at the Time, and Didn't Do It Right Away

*Therapist: What was your experience? Did you know that you were supposed to take the supplements?*

*Client*: Yeah, I've had to use them before so I know what to do.

*Therapist*: Okay, what's the next MLA question?

*Client*: Was I willing to do what was needed? (*Pauses.*) Yeah! I was.

*Therapist*: Okay, what comes next?

*Client*: Did the thought of doing what was needed or expected ever enter my mind? Yeah, I actually had to move the potassium pill bottle off my pillow, and I was going to take one.

*Therapist*: All right, so the last MLA question says, "What got in the way of doing what was needed or expected right away?"

*Client*: Ohhhh, I went to get a glass of water for the pill, and then my sister came home and she was all upset about her boyfriend and I ended up staying up until 1:00 A.M. talking with her on the sofa! By the time I went to bed, I didn't even think about it.

*Therapist*: I can see how that would happen! You had every intention to follow the protocol and you wanted to be there for your sister. That is a tough one. Do you think there is anything you could do in the future to make sure you take the supplement should something similar happen?

*Client*: Oh . . . I could have just said that I needed to take my medication. My sister is super supportive and would have been fine with me running upstairs. I actually thought about it at one time but prioritized my sister's feelings over my health. I think I need to work on that!

*Therapist*: I like that solution! Let's try to practice communicating with others and prioritizing your health then!

Often, the MLA will take you back to commitment strategies ("I knew, and didn't want to eat"). You will find yourself weaving in pros and cons ("Tell me more about why not eating in this situation was helpful for you"), devil's advocate ("Maybe you shouldn't eat ever again"), door-in-the-face/foot-in-the-door ("Oh! We need to put together a full cope ahead plan for eating when you don't want to/what do you think about using phone coaching in moments like that when you knew what to do but couldn't bring yourself to eat?"), freedom to choose in the absence of alternatives ("I mean, not eating in the face of bradycardia makes me anxious and we can't move forward like this"), and linking to prior commitments ("We agreed to work on not eating when you are medically stable. That was our one non-negotiable: to stay alive. You aren't bailing on me, are you?").

## BCA Example

Let's take a look now at the case study at the start of this chapter through the lens of a BCA. Your client reported leaving the hospital and entering a binge-purge cycle that led to another hospital admission. At your next individual session, you want to explore what happened as you felt you both had a clear plan to manage the T1 behavior from the previous session.

In order to identify the target behavior for the chain, it is very important to separate ED behaviors and not lump them together as one singular event. For example, we find many practitioners attempt to target "binge-purge behaviors" in the same chain, however, while related, these are two distinct actions. The factors that prompt and maintain the binge may not be the same as the factors that prompt and maintain the purge. These are two separate chains. When multiple symptoms are present (restricting, binge eating, purging, self-injury), use the target hierarchy to decide which to focus on in session. While the symptoms are connected (e.g., restriction increases urges to binge eat, which, in turn, increases urges to purge), you will need to prioritize which behaviors are riskiest. In our case study, the purging is causing electrolyte abnormalities. Your job will be to determine whether to target the purging or the binge episode. If the binge is what is causing the purging (e.g., without binge eating, your client wouldn't purge), then it makes sense to focus there.

There are important nuances and points to consider when a BCA is applied to ED behaviors. Perhaps most important is to remain mindful of your own biases or assumptions when it comes to treating eating, weight, and shape difficulties. Sometimes, when conducting BCAs, clinicians focus heavily on mechanical eating without targeting the emotional underpinnings. In other cases, practitioners assume that ED behaviors are simply a matter of emotion regulation and fail to target the neurometabolic drivers of the behavior.

## Points to Consider in Your Solution Analysis

For a majority of patients, food and fluid restriction sets up a strong biological drive to binge eat. Teaching your client about the restrict-binge-purge cycle is an important aspect of this work. It is also difficult to successfully eliminate binge eating without regular eating. That said, understanding the role of restriction is often complicated and multilayered. Restriction can serve many functions, one of which is to soothe an unsettled biology that includes GI distress, perceptual difficulties, and distressing sensory experiences. Restriction can also help a person navigate invalidating environments and sociocultural pressures, suppress emotions, and increase focus and attentional qualities. Your BCAs will help provide clarity for you and your client regarding the unique ways restriction is reinforced (both biologically and socially). Your solution analysis will need to take into account these specific findings rather than having generalized approaches to food restriction (e.g., everyone must begin mechanical eating right away; everyone must use a feared food hierarchy). Generalizations often miss the mark for our clients who have tried those approaches with minimal success. A client may first (or concurrently) need help to manage GI pain, tolerate distress, or learn interpersonal effectiveness skills in order for regular eating to be effective.

As we do in all chains, we help our clients move from nonspecific terms ("I felt fat") to behavioral descriptors ("I noticed a sensation of tightness from my pants on my belly"). Help your client notice when "diet culture" shows up. When your client says that they "feel fat," we may observe that statement as internalized weight bias given that "feeling fat" communicates that there is something inherently disgusting or bad about fat. In a chain, you can help your client get more specific in the links about what they mean by "feeling fat." In our experience, it usually reflects an intolerable bodily sensation. Behavioral specificity not only provides more clarity, which leads to more effective problem solving, but also removes judgment and bias from the equation, which, in and of itself, can reduce the intensity of the moment.

Breaking ED symptoms apart helps clients see that there is a distinction and one behavior does not have to lead to the next. For example, many clients tell us that they must purge if they binge eat. We have no doubt about the intensity of the urge to remove the consequences of a binge, *and* it is still possible to tolerate a binge without purging, however impossible it might feel. Separating urges from ED behaviors and helping clients see where one symptom ends and another begins is an important part of the chaining process.

Finally, tolerating fullness post-binge is a very difficult physical and emotional experience. Sometimes providers stop the chain at the target behavior and do not collect data on what happens following it. Your chain needs to include the thoughts, emotions, and actions that immediately come after the behavior. Many of our clients experience significant gastrointestinal difficulties that are exacerbated post-binge. While a focus on emotion regulation in the chain is vital, it is important to help your client observe any physical and psychological factors contributing to the behavior. Our clients need help generating solutions for how to cope with the neurobiological underpinnings of their illness.

## Summary

BCAs and MLAs are used in most MED-DBT individual therapy sessions. Together they provide a nonjudgmental and highly constructive way of exploring the variables that cause and maintain symptoms. Conversational in nature, chain analyses are collaborative and are meant to be delivered in the context of a highly dialectical and validating interaction. Chains are an effective way to approach a problem or a behavior one wants to learn more about. Early sessions will include a focus on teaching your client how to do an effective chain with the ultimate goal of supporting your client to do these more automatically. Once clients begin to recognize the patterns that drive their behaviors through BCAs and MLAs, the next step is to equip them with the tools to respond differently. In the following chapter, we explore how DBT skills, particularly when thoughtfully adapted for clients with multidiagnostic EDs, can be applied to target behavioral dyscontrol and support meaningful, sustained change.

# 15

# Considerations for Teaching DBT Skills

Much has been written about DBT skills over the past 20 years. There are several skills manuals specific to BPD, bipolar disorder, anxiety, psychosis, adolescents, and cancer treatment, just to name a few. There is also a DBT skills manual for bulimia (Astrachan-Fletcher & Maslar, 2009), an RO-DBT skills workbook (Hall et al., 2022), and two books (Safer et al., 2009, 2018) written for eating disorders. These books offer helpful examples of how to apply DBT skills to various ED difficulties. However, these texts were written for individuals with primary (e.g., not multidiagnostic) Stage 3 ED presentations and we find there are specific nuances and additions we have made over the years for our clients in Stage 1 (e.g., behavioral dyscontrol). Thus, in this chapter we share our experiences and use of DBT skills for clients with multiproblem behaviors, including common challenges and caveats. Of note, in adapting DBT, we didn't necessarily believe there needed to be new skills specific to ED treatment. Rather we needed to think about how the DBT skills were applied to our treatment targets. Most of the research to date on the effectiveness of DBT skills has been done on Linehan's original skills (1993), not on the adaptations that have come later.

## Considerations When Getting Started

Teaching "by the book" often means that practitioners are using the exact handouts, examples, and exercises from Linehan's (2025a, 2025b) *DBT Skills Training Manual* and *DBT Skills Training Handouts and Worksheets.* While it is essential to know the concepts and methods of teaching DBT skills, many of the skills as originally written were not designed for those with eating disorders, and in some cases can be problematic (e.g., teaching clients to use the temperature skill to drop blood pressure and heart rate when they are already medically unstable). On the other hand, we have observed teams trying to offer DBT skills in non-adherent ways (e.g., not sticking to the protocol, drifting from skills teaching into process groups, and sometimes removing entire skill sections from their classes for fear they are too triggering). These choices often come from a well-intentioned place: Clinicians are trying to protect clients from distress, accommodate trauma histories, or avoid reinforcing ED behaviors. However, when skills are removed, watered down, or replaced with loosely related content, the treatment loses its coherence, and clients are left without the full range of tools needed to build a life worth living.

Rather than removing skill sections entirely, we recommend adapting how they are introduced and processed. For example, if your team is concerned that the Distress Tolerance module could be triggering due to the use of cold exposure or intense exercise in the TIPP (*T*emperature, *I*ntense exercise, *P*aced breathing, and *P*rogressive muscle relaxation) skills, the solution is not to avoid teaching these skills, but to offer clinical nuance when introducing them. Teams can proactively flag potential medical concerns (e.g., bradycardia, electrolyte instability), validate the emotional and physical impact of these exercises, and collaboratively identify safe substitutions or modifications. Ultimately, we encourage teams to stay adherent to the spirit and structure of DBT while finding developmentally and medically appropriate ways to teach the skills. The goal is not to dilute the material but to make it accessible, safe, and effective for this population.

A common question we are asked is whether MED-DBT clients can be integrated into standard DBT skills groups or if they need their own group. Generally, our clients do very well in standard DBT groups and we don't separate them from other clients who are learning the skills for their unique reasons. That said, it is important that skills group facilitators are teaching skills in a way that challenges weight bias and includes application to food, meals, body image, weight stabilization, and neurobiological differences that underlie EDs. In the same way that we are all working on ensuring that skills delivery is accessible, anti-racist, and inclusive in terms of neurodiversity, gender, and culture, the inclusion of ED education and knowledge is essential. Given the overlap between EDs, emotion regulation difficulties, and trauma, there may be far more people in your skills groups than you realize suffering with an ED, but undiagnosed.

As noted in Chapter 11, one of the ways weight bias shows up in healthcare spaces is in the way offices and group rooms are designed, such as chairs with armrests or only providing smaller-sized chairs that are not accessible to those in larger bodies. Design your group rooms to be accommodating and affirming for all body shapes and sizes so that clients can easily move around the table and chairs and can feel safe with respect to the seating options. Images, artwork, and magazines that promote thin bodies or Eurocentric beauty ideals can be replaced with more culturally and body-diverse materials that make your commitment to anti-diet culture clear.

Finally, consider your client's medical and physical status and be prepared for slower change. Clients with Stage 1 EDs may be suffering from cognitive difficulties (e.g., attention, memory, processing speed, language, perception) secondary to malnourishment, physical pain due to GI discomfort, and substantive body image distress. There are times when apparent competence shows up and clinicians assume their clients have the skills to manage. Take for example a client who is highly driven, focused on pleasing others, and perfectionistic in such a way that they can be highly articulate or achieve high grades or career accomplishments. You might tell the client that they are "so smart" and "so capable" (because they are in some domains at some times) but miss that they need help in ways that others often fail to see. For these reasons, learning new skills may take longer than other clients who are not struggling with malnourishment. Repetition and ongoing practice can be especially helpful.

## Teaching Skills in MED-DBT

In this section, we outline tips and strategies for teaching skills to your clients. In general, we do not modify the original DBT skills handouts and worksheets as the fundamental principle of each skill remains the same in MED-DBT. There are definitely examples or phrases in the 2015 manual that are not consistent with a weight-inclusive stance or that will trigger some of your clients (e.g., "can you notice your body hanging off your bones," scripts including noticing that "the chair doesn't tell you are too fat or too thin"). We take a dialectical stance about these sorts of things rather than decide ahead of time not to use them.

### Mindfulness Skills

#### Teaching States of Mind

Often the tendency is to place "ED mind" within the "emotion mind" sphere when applied to EDs. In emotion mind, our clients are driven by affective states, and the faculties of logic and reason are either less available or subordinate to emotion. While ED behaviors may well be represented as a function of emotion mind for some clients, some of the time, it is also true that ED behaviors exist in "reasonable mind," where reliance on excessive habits, tasks, pragmatics, and rules dominates. In reasonable mind, access to values and emotional data is inaccessible and/or less salient.

Sometimes there is a tendency to want to categorize our clients as being either one dominant way or the other. To date, that is not our experience as our clients, who can be quite overcontrolled in many circumstances ("reasonable mind") can quickly become ruled by emotions when having to eat food or gain weight. While we work on activating wise mind with our clients, we also help them observe and describe the inevitable shifts in states of mind that define their experience. Putting words to this experience without judgment, exploring the function of those shifts biologically and emotionally, and linking the oscillation to the adapted biosocial theory is incredibly helpful for you and your client. Questions to explore with your client might include the following:

- How does being in reasonable mind (and relying on habits, rules, and logic) help you cope with your symptoms?
- How does emotion mind (acting quickly on feelings, urges) help you cope?
- How does emotion mind show up at meals? What about reasonable mind? Would wise mind show up differently?
- What would a wise mind response to an urge to purge/binge eat/restrict sound like for you?

### "What" and "How" Skills

In addition to all the ways we teach the "what" and "how" skills per Linehan (2025a, 2025b), there are important things to consider or focus on when teaching this skill set to your clients.

- *Observe.* We can help slow things down and be more present (and therefore more able to change the things we want to) when we can accurately observe our experiences. We ask our clients to observe emotions that arise at a meal or when looking in the mirror, urges to body check or body avoid, thoughts that are present when someone comments on their weight or eating behavior. As in standard DBT, we are working to cultivate awareness of emotions/thoughts/images around the ED and to allow them to come and go without attaching to them (nonstick mind) or pushing them away.

- *Describe.* The ability to accurately represent experience opens up many options for our clients (e.g., more effective coping plans, improved communication about needs), *and* our clients often avoid talking about body and eating or do so with substantial judgment. We use the describe skill to help our clients put words to their physical sensations, including pain and discomfort, their perceptual and sensory experiences around food and body, and the presence of weight bias/diet culture ("I noticed diet culture entered the room when my doctor was happy that I lost weight.").
- *Participate.* Cultivating the ability to be fully immersed in an experience is a potent skill and can be a powerful antidote to loneliness, body distress, and self-consciousness. For example, it's nearly impossible to ruminate about the next meal or body image when a client is completely absorbed in painting a mural or fully engaged in laughing with a friend or playing with a pet. However, our clients can overuse this skill by throwing themselves excessively into the experience of eating a meal or overexercising in a way that exacerbates the ED and their emotion regulation capacities. Yet, when our clients hone the skill of being in a moment effectively and without judgment, this can have far-reaching benefits. We work with our clients to generate ideas for using this skill both on a daily basis and in difficult circumstances (e.g., at meals, at the beach in a bathing suit).
- *Non-judgment.* A powerhouse of a skill for our clients, practicing a nonjudgmental stance toward the body, food, and the diet-centric environment we live in helps to reduce emotional intensity and increases the likelihood of acting from our values. Self-criticism, self-hatred, and body loathing/despair are disproportionately high in our clients. We worked with a client who would enter our skills group room with announcements such as "make way for the fat woman" or "look out, large object coming through." Seeing this as an opportunity, we asked her if she noticed this pattern of entering a space with judgment. She replied, "Yes, I do this everywhere because it's true and everybody thinks it anyway." She described that this had become a way to protect herself "by saying what others were already thinking" so nobody could beat her to it: This made her feel like she had some power over it.

Using the practice of non-judgment, the therapist offered an invitation: "What would it be like if today was the last day you spoke about your body judgmentally?" It was an emotional moment. The client became tearful and sat down at the table. "I don't know if I can do that," she said, "but I wish I could." Sitting down next to her, the therapist said, "I know it won't be easy because it has this protective quality to it, and I wonder if we could try it as an experiment and see what that is like for you?" Ironically, it did not take long for the client to feel empowered by the stance that she was standing up to diet culture and not apologizing for her body.

- *One-mindfully*. Focusing on doing one thing at a time has helped our clients cope during meals ("Just this one bite") and manage body distress ("Right now, in this changing room, I can feel my breath and the texture of the fabric"). We use one-mindfully to teach our clients how to be just in this singular moment rather than being attached to the past or playing out the future ("I won't be able to handle dinner out with friends tonight, so I need to plan where and when to purge"). We encourage you to talk with your client about how to be fully focused on the present moment in a way that doesn't emphasize ED thoughts and feelings. Some of our clients are very skilled at hyperfocusing on their bodies or on food in the moment. Remind your client that focusing on just this moment is more than the body or the food, it is a focus on all the sensory elements that make up this moment in time (e.g., the feel of the cushions beneath you, the sounds of music coming from your phone, the sight of trees outside your window budding in the spring air).

  It is important to note that sometimes this skill is interpreted as a "green light" for mindful eating. While helpful for people with a primary diagnosis of binge-eating disorder, mindful eating is not something we recommend for our clients in Stage 1 who are working on medical stability and stabilizing food intake and weight (Marek et al., 2013). Mindful eating for someone who is emotionally sensitive, in behavioral instability, and may have sensory and perceptual experiences related to food and digestion is often more than they can manage without more skills around them.

- *Effectiveness*. Approaching a situation with the goal of being effective rather than "right" can be hard to navigate. A big focus in MED-DBT is figuring out how to help our clients get their needs met effectively in weight-biased environments or with healthcare professionals who lack ED training. This might involve strategizing about how to get lab work done when the family doctor says it is unnecessary or helping your client manage a difficult living situation that exacerbates the ED and suicidal thinking. Being effective is also important when talking about eating. For example, eating only lettuce at lunch is not effective for preventing binge/purge behaviors later. Likewise, choosing the safe item on the menu might not be effective for feeling satisfied.

## Distress Tolerance Skills

Designed to help your client get through short-term crises without making things worse, distress tolerance (DT) skills are divided into two main categories: distraction skills and acceptance strategies. Many clients will acknowledge suicide and self-injurious behaviors as crises but may not identify ED behaviors in the same way. Therefore, it is useful to discuss with your client the types of ED-specific scenarios that they experience for which DT skills will be beneficial. This can include urges to purge, tolerating fullness and physical discomfort after a binge episode, getting on the scale in the office, dealing with GI distress, attending a medical appointment to get labs done, eating alone, eating with others, or feeling the tightness of clothing. It is incredibly important to prepare clients for the fact that the skill may work, *and* you may still feel awful. As an example, a client with bulimia came into session very angry and tired after what he described as an awfully long night trying to manage urges to binge and purge.

*Client*: These skills are so stupid! I've barely slept! They don't work. I am done with the DBT crap.

*Therapist*: Okay, can you tell me what happened?!

*Client*: Yeah! I practiced the three skills we talked about after dinner and they didn't work. My urges were through the roof!

*Therapist*: I appreciate that you tried to use the skills like we talked about. Did you end up bingeing and purging then?

*Client*: "Use your skills, use your skills . . ." (*Rolls his eyes.*) Nobody understands that this isn't helping!

*Therapist*: I am 1,000% seeing how exacerbated you are.

*Client*: I was up until 4:30 this morning just using my skills. This is dumb.

*Therapist*: Wow, that is a long night for sure. Is that when you had symptoms?

*Client*: What?!

*Therapist*: I am just trying to figure out where the symptoms came in last night/this morning?

*Client*: I didn't have any symptoms.

*Therapist*: Wait, what?

*Client*: No, I was up all night doing activities and using ice and writing out pros and cons. You should see my bedroom! It's all warm ice packs and crumbled up balls of paper, and some decent crocheted scarves . . . !

*Therapist*: But no binge–purge behaviors?

*(Client and therapist looking at each other in a moment of silence.)*

*Client*: No . . . no binge–purge behaviors.

*Therapist*: Not at all trying to sound like a jerk, but . . . are you telling me that the skills worked!?

*Client*: (*Laughs and collapses onto the sofa.*) Well shit, if that is the skills working, that's one hell of a ride!

*Therapist*: (*smiling*) Yeah, it can go like that some days. Right now, your purging is almost always landing you back in the hospital, so I am going to take this as a massive win on your part. Don't get me wrong, it's hard and I wish it was faster or smoother somehow. It's another dialectical tension: The skills can work *and* it can feel really intense to ride out urges. That is why we can't just rely on DT skills. We need them to prevent us from making things worse but they won't solve all of your problems.

As you will do with all DBT skills, showing clients how the skills apply to their experience and giving ED-relevant examples is very important. In the DT module, some examples include the following:

- *STOP skill.* Described as the "portal skill," the STOP skill is the precursor to all the other skills. Encourage your client to STOP when they notice the urge to body check, skip out on lunch, or avoid going to the doctor.
- *Pros/cons.* Have your client write out the pros and cons of purging, exercising, chewing and spitting *before* deciding whether to act on the urge.
- *Wise mind ACCEPTS.* Have your client write out (and gather the materials needed) for a complete ACCEPTS protocol to be used at meals.

- *IMPROVE the moment.* Help your client plan out an entire IMPROVE protocol to be used when they are on bed rest, while sitting in the lab waiting room, or when having to attend a family meal.
- *TIPP skills* (Temperature, Intense exercise, Paced breathing, and Progressive muscle relaxation). These are powerful DT techniques designed to rapidly reduce emotional arousal by shifting physiological responses. They are often the "go-to" interventions for managing acute emotional distress due to their ability to quickly change body chemistry. However, in the context of MED-DBT, these skills must be used with caution. For instance, placing one's face in cold water to activate the dive reflex may sound harmless, but this technique lowers heart rate and blood pressure rapidly—something that can be dangerous for clients already struggling to maintain medical stability. Similarly, paced breathing can further reduce heart rate, which is problematic for clients with bradycardia. (We once had a client whose smartwatch alerted her during group that her heart rate had dropped into the low 40s after practicing paced breathing.) Intense exercise, another component of TIPP, may also pose serious risks: For some clients it exacerbates medical instability, while for others it reinforces ED-related compulsions. In all cases, the use of TIPP skills requires thoughtful clinical judgment and individualization to ensure safety and effectiveness.

  Sometimes we are asked whether the TIPP handout should be removed altogether when teaching DBT skills. We do not agree with that approach. The reality is that our clients are exposed to these strategies online and from other therapists, and we would rather have conversations about staying safe and being effective rather than avoiding the topic. We ask our clients to get clearance from their physicians before using these skills. If there is no medical instability, these skills should be used as normal.
- *Self-soothing.* Designed to increase one's ability to cope, these skills take on a particular meaning among those living with EDs, and it is not uncommon for our clients to avoid using them. Talk with your clients about how interoceptive awareness difficulties interfere with connecting to the senses and discuss the way in which common ED sensory and perceptual differences help or hinder one's ability to self-soothe. Without these discussions, there is an assumption that clients "should" be able to see, feel, hear, smell, and taste in a particular way. While some clients can find soothing with the senses helpful over time, others

may not habituate even with practice. Some of our clients with oral sensitivities will struggle to find taste soothing and others will have fears about enjoying food or associating regulation with calories and taste. On the other hand, some clients are already using food and taste to soothe themselves. With respect to the latter, acknowledge the wisdom of using this skill ("food IS soothing") and explore whether your client is overusing it to the exclusion of other self-regulation strategies. This is an opportunity to help them build a more robust repertoire of self-soothing skills.

- *Radical acceptance.* Developing the ability to accept reality for what it is (e.g., the genetics of weight, biological drivers of appetite) rather than fighting reality for what it isn't (e.g., being able to get rid of the desire to eat) is not easy for anyone, and yet is a skill for everyday life. To live is to encounter many things that we don't like and can't control. The acceptance strategies in DBT are essential to emotion regulation and provide guidance on how to live with (rather than against) the aspects of our lives that we don't want to accept. We agree that pain is inevitable but that suffering ensues when we judge, resist, and reject that pain.

So, what does this mean for our clients? As we do in standard DBT, it means accepting things we cannot change in the present moment, particularly when struggling against them only causes more suffering. In the ED context, this also involves radically acknowledging the genetics of body weight and the biology of appetite regulation without judgment or attempts to change it. It means accepting that you have an ED and recognizing the impact it has on your life without dismissal or disallowance.

Take, for example, our client who worked incredibly hard to stabilize her health only to realize that recovery meant living in a larger body ("I cannot radically accept that this is where my body wants to be! This is so unfair!"). In the context of a highly validating space, the therapist also maintained an unwavering focus on helping the client to "turn the mind" from diet culture. They practiced willing hands and half-smiling when she wore clothing that increased body image distress. They looked at the pros and cons of fighting versus accepting her biology. It took time and patience. Slowly, over the course of treatment, the client was able to access a more compassionate, willing, and accepting stance toward her biology, the prominence of diet culture in her environment, and the biological drivers of her ED (e.g., perceptual difficulties, interoceptive differences). In time, her ability to cope ahead and to manage difficult situations improved in proportion to her practice of radical acceptance.

## Emotion Regulation Skills

Linehan's Emotion Regulation module begins by educating clients about the purpose and function of emotions, as well as the factors that make emotional regulation particularly difficult. In MED-DBT, this material is adapted to reflect the unique challenges faced by individuals with EDs. Specifically, we expand the discussion of biological vulnerability to include the effects of malnourishment, dysregulated metabolism, and the neurobiological consequences of chronic ED behaviors. These additions help clients better understand why their emotional experiences may feel especially intense, unpredictable, or difficult to manage, and why traditional strategies for emotion regulation may not have been effective in the past. When introducing this material, we encourage a collaborative and non-shaming approach that helps clients connect their physiological experiences with their emotional ones, laying the groundwork for both compassion and change.

### Teaching Clients about Their Emotions

Observing, describing, and managing all emotions are vital goals of the MED-DBT model. As in standard DBT, we teach our clients how to identify primary and secondary emotions with accuracy and compassion. We have noticed, however, that emotions such as disgust, envy, shame, and jealousy get less "air time" compared to their more popular counterparts (e.g., anxiety, anger, and sadness), even though they are often central experiences for our clients. Given the link to eating and body experiences, regularly discussing the role of disgust and envy will be important in this work.

Another notable consideration relates to the impact of malnourishment and interoceptive awareness difficulties on emotional identification. In 2015, Linehan (p. 341) noted that "sometimes the problem with emotion is that you cannot sense your body and its changes. To regulate emotions, you have to be skilled in sensing your body." But what happens when, like many of our clients, a person is unable to accurately sense their body due to biological differences in sensation and perception? How does the absence of adequate nourishment—and the muting effects of starvation—interfere with the ability to connect to internal cues and bodily sensations? What may seem like a helpful suggestion (e.g., asking your client to check in with their body to identify emotions) can, when delivered without nuance, feel ableist or invalidating. These practices must be adapted to reflect your client's unique sensory, perceptual, and nutritional realities.

We recommend weaving in psychoeducation about how malnourishment and interoceptive awareness difficulties can interfere with emotional detection. Rather than assuming clients will "figure it out" by reviewing standard DBT materials on their own, take a collaborative and curious stance. Work together to experiment with different ways of noticing and labeling emotions and explore which strategies feel most accessible and effective for your client. Be prepared for this process to unfold more slowly than it might in standard DBT, especially given the physiological and perceptual barriers many clients with EDs experience. Patience, flexibility, and validation are key.

When teaching clients how to identify and describe emotions, we recommend expanding the language and examples typically used in standard DBT to better reflect the lived experiences of individuals with EDs. For instance, when exploring the emotion of disgust, it can be helpful to include ED-specific prompting events such as food texture, oral sensitivities, food odors, or body image-related triggers, elements that are often absent in more general descriptions. Including thoughts and action urges that are commonly linked to these ED-related experiences helps clients feel seen and supported and increases the relevance and accessibility of emotion education in this population.

### Checking the Facts

Teaching your client how to determine if an emotion is justified by evaluating factual evidence is an important skill set. When checking the facts related to ED behaviors, it is important to use your knowledge of weight stigma and to be aware of your beliefs and biases about eating as you navigate these discussions. We don't want to perpetuate the invalidating environment by invalidating the valid! For example, you may be inclined to challenge your client's statement that pasta is disgusting: "but pasta is so soft and easier to eat!" you might say, however, disgust may make sense for someone with ARFID who has particular sensory differences. Instead, we might respond by saying, "I wonder if the experience of disgust is related to some of the sensory differences we talked about? It may be a fact that you experience pasta and other foods with a more pronounced reaction of disgust." That being said, it may be that once the facts are checked, the primary emotion is fear rather than disgust or there may be circumstances in which the intensity or duration of disgust may not fit the facts. Your job is to explore how an emotion like disgust arises in the context of understanding the genetic underpinnings of an ED. We also must stay dialectical: It makes sense that disgust is triggered in this scenario *and* it may need to be targeted when it severely interferes with food and fluid intake and/or quality of life. Similarly, if the emotion is fear and the fear is of weight gain I might need to check the facts about whether or not this particular meal will make me gain weight and if it is true that this meal might make me gain weight then I need to also practice acceptance or opposite action and link up to my bigger goals of why I am exposing myself to this meal in the first place.

Checking the facts around body image concerns is another area that can easily become invalidating in the absence of a weight-neutral lens. Traditional ED models encourage clients to evaluate the strength of their beliefs using thought records or by charting body weight to "test out" beliefs (e.g., noticing big emotional or cognitive swings in body image distress without related fluctuations in weight). While helpful in some circumstances, these approaches can sometimes communicate that one's thoughts and fears about weight gain are merely "distortions" or exaggerated beliefs. Your client may need to gain weight *and* gaining weight might have significant relational, physical, and emotional consequences. Take, for example, a client who experienced weight and shape-based bullying throughout elementary and high school and whose family and friends responded more positively to them when they lost weight. Gaining weight in Western society can be scary and sometimes unsafe for people (e.g., physician refusal to treat if above a certain BMI, increased bullying at higher weights). It is also true, given the neurometabolic underpinnings of EDs, that weight gain can be experienced as very uncomfortable and can cause a number of distressing physical sensations. Therefore, it is important not to assume that all fears of weight gain or all sensory/perceptual experiences are simply cognitive "errors." We wish to reemphasize the fact that we are all influenced by diet culture and have internalized much of that philosophy over the course of our lives. This will impact your work. Delivering MED-DBT comes with the expectation that you are doing your own work to uncover and challenge diet culture beliefs and attitudes. The more you lean into this, the more adept you will be at navigating the dialectical tensions in these challenging discussions!

### Acting Opposite at Meals

It is often the case that our clients are simply told to act opposite as *the* skill to use at meals (e.g., asking your client to act opposite by picking up their fork or taking another bite). While hugely important, it can come across as "Regardless of your emotion, you just need to eat," which is a message they have heard ad nauseum and can increase distress. In other words, it isn't acting opposite so you can eat because you have an ED. It is acting opposite to (insert emotion, such as disgust) because it is intense and you want to reduce that affective state. It is also true that if your client believes a food is disgusting, their emotions will increase when exposed to that food and they will likely need more coaching to address this.

### Myths and Beliefs about Emotions

Conversations about emotional myths can be incredibly powerful for clients, especially those who have long felt invalidated, misunderstood, or unsure about how emotions "should" work. In our experience, inviting clients to identify and challenge their personal beliefs about emotions opens the door to increased insight, compassion, and cognitive flexibility. These discussions can also serve as a turning point in treatment, especially when clients begin to see how rigid beliefs have contributed to emotional avoidance, shame, or reliance on the ED and co-occurring symptoms as primary ways to manage emotions.

While many clients endorse common cultural myths (e.g., "Showing emotion is a sign of weakness," or "If I feel something, I have to act on it"), those living with EDs often endorse additional beliefs that are shaped by malnourishment and diet culture. Together with our clients, we have compiled and explored ED-specific myths and beliefs such as the following:

- "In order for my emotions to be taken seriously, I have to lose weight."
- "Emotions can only be managed through the ED."
- "My ED is the only part of me that makes sense emotionally."
- "I have to be better/stronger/more pure than others."
- "I cannot eat when I feel disgust."

These beliefs are often deeply entrenched and may have been reinforced by providers, family members, or treatment environments. Exploring them with your client can offer opportunities to validate how these beliefs developed while also questioning whether they still serve the client's long-term life worth living goals. It is often helpful to explore the function of these beliefs and what emotions or experiences they help the client avoid, control, or explain. We encourage you to be curious and collaborative, inviting your clients to generate their own myths and reflect on where they came from, how they've helped, and what the costs have been. The goal isn't to quickly replace these beliefs, but to bring them into the light and explore alternatives that are more flexible, compassionate, and sustainable.

### PLEASE Skills

In the early days of implementing MED-DBT, we noticed that some colleagues were removing the PLEASE skills from their groups altogether, believing them to be incompatible with ED treatment. We disagree! The PLEASE skills are highly relevant to ED care and offer a valuable framework for helping clients understand how extremes in eating, sleeping, exercise, and managing physical illness can impact emotion regulation. The PLEASE skills also provide an effective, nonjudgmental way to begin conversations with clients about the overwhelming and often contradictory (mis)information they receive from social media and broader cultural messages related to health and eating. Rather than removing the skill, we advocate for adapting it, as seen in Table 15.1.

## Interpersonal Effectiveness Skills

The Interpersonal Effectiveness (IE) module is a core component of DBT, offering clients concrete tools to clarify their goals in relationships, express needs, maintain self-respect, and navigate social dynamics more effectively. In MED-DBT, we retain the core structure of this module while thoughtfully expanding it to reflect the specific challenges faced by clients with EDs. These include not only the emotional and behavioral vulnerabilities common in DBT populations but also the social, physiological, and cultural complexities unique to ED recovery.

It is often the case that our clients engage in behaviors that are triggered and maintained by interpersonal circumstances. Similar to clients in standard DBT, they may have difficulty accurately identifying and expressing their relational needs, struggle to say no or assert themselves, may be conflict avoidant, and may prematurely end relationships or hang on to unhealthy connections for too long. These difficulties are compounded by the emotional and cognitive effects of malnourishment, internalized weight stigma, and repeated experiences of invalidation, particularly in healthcare or family systems. IE skills are also necessary to manage ED recovery. For instance, navigating meal planning and timing (e.g., I need to eat now rather than later), social outings (e.g., can we go to a different restaurant?), and

**TABLE 15.1 Supporting Emotion Regulation through Tailored PLEASE Skills**

| | Linehan's (2025) wording | MED-DBT additions |
|---|---|---|
| *P*hysical | Being sick lowers your resistance to negative emotions. The healthier you can become, the better able you will be to regulate your emotions. Many individuals fear going to a physician or do not have the behavioral regulation to get themselves to doctor appointments. Others do not have the self-regulation to take prescribed medications (either psychotropics or general medication). | Important to explore possibly value on being the most ill, neglect, and disgust of the body in general, and overall tolerance for being sick among those with EDs. Explore possibly the role of anosognosia on the ability to detect physical illness and pain. |
| *L*imit Social Media Use | Originally, the "L" was part of "PL" = PhysicaL illness. | Increased use of social media is linked to worsening emotion regulation and body image disturbances. Increases access to diet culture and inaccurate messages about food, eating, and body weight. |
| *E*ating in Balance | Try to eat the amounts and kinds of foods that help you feel good—not too much or too little. When and how often you eat and your daily eating routine can be especially important for some individuals. Stay away from food that makes you feel overly emotional. | Important for our clients to learn to eat regularly/"by-the-clock," and to refrain from dieting/restricting food or fluid intake. Emphasis is placed on teaching clients how to eat in ways that support other co-occurring physical conditions (e.g., migraines, epilepsy) and sensory difficulties. |
| *A*void Mood-Altering Substances | Alcohol and drugs, like certain foods, can lower resistance to negative emotions. Stay off mood-altering substances. Use alcohol in moderation (if at all). | Important to assess and educate about the role of stimulant medications, caffeine, cannabis use, or other substances that may suppress hunger cues, increase grogginess/missing meals due to fatigue, and/or facilitate weight loss. |
| Balanced *S*leep | Try to get the amount of sleep that helps you feel good—not too much or too little, usually between 7 and 9 hours. Keep to a consistent sleep schedule, especially if you are having difficulty sleeping. | Sleep disturbances are common in those with EDs and uniquely linked to malnourishment, over/under exercise, purging, and so on. |

(*Continued*)

**TABLE 15.1 (Continued)**

| | Linehan's (2025) wording | MED-DBT additions |
|---|---|---|
| *E*xercise | Aerobic exercise, done consistently, is an antidepressant. Do some sort of exercise five to seven days per week. Try to build up to 20 minutes of exercise each time. | Some clients will need to learn how to take breaks from exercise (e.g., scheduling rest days) and/ or develop more balanced ways of engaging in movement. In some cases, a temporary break from activity, or even prescribed bedrest, may be required as part of treatment. Additionally, many clients will need coaching and support to reintroduce exercise in a non-eating disorder-driven way. |

*Note*. From *DBT Skills Training Manual, Revised Edition* by Marsha M. Linehan. Copyright © 2025 The Guilford Press. Reprinted by permission.

being able to assert oneself without aggression, passivity, or relying on ED behaviors to increase the chance of needs being met (e.g., stating "I need your help" instead of saying "I hope I die from starvation" in order to be seen/heard). In this section, we provide examples of ways to enhance the interpersonal effectiveness module for your clients:

## Enhancing Interpersonal Skills for ED-Relevant Contexts

### WHAT GETS IN THE WAY?

In standard DBT, clients explore how indecision, emotions, environmental obstacles, and worrying thoughts interfere with relational goals. In MED-DBT, we extend this exploration to include the following:

- *Inadequate nutrition,* which impairs cognitive, emotional, and physical difficulties that impact relationships, intimacy, connectedness, and accurate communication.
- *Weight stigma and diet culture.* It is very challenging to get one's needs met in environments that are dominated by weight bias and diet culture (e.g., asking your parents to buy foods from your meal plan that they view as "junk food," talking with your family about why you eat breakfast when they engage in intermittent fasting, asking your doctor for lab work when they tell you your weight is fine).
- *Invalidating systems,* such as healthcare settings or family dynamics that dismiss or pathologize clients' experiences, reinforce silence or withdrawal, or perpetuate outdated or misinformed views of EDs—make it especially difficult for clients to express their needs. For example, a

client may struggle to advocate for necessary lab work when a doctor insists they can't have an ED "because they are still menstruating."

### Beliefs That Interfere with Effectiveness

Many of the beliefs that interfere with IE skills for those with EDs are valid and a reflection of the dominant weight-phobic, diet-centered culture. Therefore, it is essential not to label a rational thought (e.g., "I am afraid to gain weight and increase chances of being bullied at school again") as a myth. That said, clients often internalize beliefs that limit their ability to engage skillfully in relationships. These include the following:

- "Someone in a larger body should stay as quiet as possible, not rock the boat."
- "People won't take me seriously if I have gained weight."
- "My needs are only valid when I am at a low weight."
- "I deserve to be punished for my body or eating behavior."
- "I have to be confident in my body image before I can make requests or say no."
- "If I look ill, people will approach me, and I will receive more intimacy."

Rather than disputing these beliefs outright, we approach them dialectically: validating the context in which they arose, while also exploring whether they are helping or hindering movement toward a life worth living.

### Applying Interpersonal Effectiveness Skills in ED Contexts

In the section of the module related to "obtaining objectives skillfully," several important considerations arise when working with clients in MED-DBT. While the core DBT strategies, such as DEAR MAN, GIVE, and FAST, are essential, their application often requires modification or expansion to reflect the complex realities of ED recovery.

- *Clarifying needs.* This can be a particularly difficult exercise for our clients, especially given the effects of malnourishment and interoceptive awareness difficulties. Many clients are deeply disconnected from knowing what they need, not only due to biology but also due to their learning history (e.g., chronic suppression, dismissal, or avoidance of needs). These factors must be acknowledged and thoughtfully integrated into discussions about interpersonal effectiveness. Without this, clients may feel shame or confusion about their inability to articulate what they want or ask for support.

- *Teaching DEAR MAN, GIVE, and FAST with ED-specific relevance.* While you'll teach these skills as outlined in standard DBT, we recommend using examples that reflect your clients' lived experiences. This helps with skill generalization and reduces the risk of invalidation through abstract or nonrelevant scenarios. Some useful examples include the following:
    - ☐ Asking a parent to purchase food for a meal plan
    - ☐ Telling a family member not to comment on your weight
    - ☐ Saying no when friends invite you to the gym
    - ☐ Refusing to be weighed outside of consensual ED treatment
    - ☐ Asking coworkers to refrain from diet culture talk at work

## Summary

DBT skills training is a fundamental part of the MED-DBT model and an integral part of our client's recovery. As with all aspects of MED-DBT, skills are taught from an affirming and weight-inclusive philosophy. While Linehan's original skills do not require a major overhaul, we recognize that the standard DBT material was not written with EDs in mind. As such, this chapter has highlighted key adaptations and clinical considerations that reflect ED current science and lived experience.

It is essential that you remain up-to-date and willing to add or modify skills with the evolving research on EDs. Skills must be delivered in a way that acknowledges your client's physiological reality, reinforces medical safety, and attends to the social and cultural contexts they are navigating, including weight bias and diet culture. ED-specific examples help clients generalize what they learn, while adaptations to language, pacing, and expectations allow space for the unique challenges your clients face (e.g., difficulties with interoception).

Of course, teaching skills in session is only part of the equation. True mastery happens when clients are supported to use those skills in the moments they need them most. In the next chapter, we explore how phone coaching serves as a critical tool for real-time skill application, helping clients generalize what they've learned to their everyday lives. You'll learn how to adapt standard DBT coaching practices to the unique needs of clients with multidiagnostic EDs, and how to navigate the common challenges that arise in this process.

# 16

# Adaptations for Phone Coaching

Phone coaching is an extremely powerful and essential component of comprehensive DBT. The ability to help clients interrupt behaviors and apply skills in the heat of a moment is one of the most potent interventions in DBT. The inclusion of phone coaching as a core modality was based on the observation that clients with pervasive emotion and interpersonal difficulties required more than once/week contact with their therapist in order to practice new skills. Phone coaching also addresses the issue of people learning a skill in one context (e.g., a therapist's office) when they are likely regulated, and then being asked to use the skill in other contexts when they are less likely to be regulated (e.g., a client learns the STOP skill in session, but then needs to apply it at home when facing the urge to binge after an argument with a parent or partner). Phone coaching allows us to help our clients practice skills in a variety of environments. As in standard DBT, phone coaching in MED-DBT tends to elicit a fair amount of anxiety and apprehension for many clinicians (which needs to be targeted in order to effectively apply the full MED-DBT model). In this chapter, we describe the rationale for using phone coaching with our clients, important adaptations to the standard DBT coaching protocol, and provide examples of how to use phone coaching effectively.

## Why Phone Coaching in MED-DBT?

You know those sessions that go so well? You and your client are on the same page, and there is a plan to use skills when the urge to purge or restrict comes up. Your client reports feeling motivated by the plan. You are good to go! And then, one week later at the next session, your client tells you all the ways the plan fell apart. You and your client might feel deflated, anxious, or frustrated.

It is often the case, given the many struggles our clients are managing, that even the best-laid plans in an individual session are not easy to implement outside of that session in real-life circumstances. Intense emotions, distressing thoughts, unexpected life events all collide to keep our clients off balance and unable to use new strategies without more support. Phone coaching provides a lifeline to the stability of the treatment so your client can stay afloat by learning to apply skills in the moment.

In standard DBT, phone coaching is primarily used to reduce and interrupt suicidal and self-injurious behaviors and to help manage other situations that lead to targeted behaviors (e.g., interpersonal distress, loneliness, other impulsive urges). Research has shown that clients in DBT who regularly use phone coaching have better clinical outcomes (Edwards et al., 2021). To that end, the goals of phone coaching are as follows:

- To generalize skills to the client's day-to-day life
- To interrupt urges for targeted behavior
- To manage a crisis effectively
- To repair/soothe a therapy rupture

In MED-DBT, phone coaching plays the same essential role and has been extended to account for ED urges and behaviors. While ED behaviors may appear to be similar to usual DBT targets (e.g., suicide, self-injury, substance use), they are different in important ways. For example, phone coaching often focuses on ways to remove, reduce, or abstain from triggers and prompting events, whereas in EDs we often have to help clients move toward and increase exposure to the distressing stimuli—namely, eating and body experiencing. Unlike symptoms that come and go, our clients have to navigate food and fluid intake multiple times per day while learning ways to live more peacefully in their bodies. In our experience, many clinicians feel unsure how to use phone coaching effectively, resulting in either its removal altogether or increased burnout (and lack of fidelity to the model) due to receiving multiple calls per day.

The first step to effective phone coaching is orienting your client to the function and parameters of between-session contact. In addition to the rationale we provide in standard DBT, we highlight that phone coaching in MED-DBT helps clients do the following:

- Stay on track with meal plans
- Reduce urges to purge, binge eat, exercise, and so on.
- Maintain medical stability
- Increase ability to tolerate/radically accept body sensations
- Apply skills to reduce vulnerability to diet culture
- Use interpersonal effectiveness skills at mealtimes
- Help with meal completion

## The Next Meal/Snack Rule

The most significant adaptation to phone coaching in MED-DBT involves adjusting the 24-hour rule in favor of the next meal/snack rule (NM/S). Phone coaching is designed to be offered *before* your client acts on an urge. You want your client to call you as a preventative strategy to practice the skills they are learning in group in the heat of the moment. Phone coaching in standard DBT is suspended for 24 hours if a client engages in suicide or self-injurious behavior in order to remove the possibility of reinforcement through more warmth, compassion, or time from you immediately following a target behavior (Linehan, 1993; Ben-Porath, 2014; Chapman, 2019). Similarly, our clients have histories of receiving the care and attention they need only when they are very ill (e.g., "My mother only takes time off work to sit with me and paint our nails together when I am on the inpatient unit") with a removal of that attention or warmth when symptoms are less prominent.

Due to significant morbidity and mortality rates in our clients, and the fact that they need to eat throughout the day, the 24-hour rule has been modified in MED-DBT. As outlined in previous texts (Limbrunner et al., 2011; Bhatnager et al., 2017; Wisniewski & Ben-Porath, 2005), removing the therapist for 24 hours after a client engages in an ED behavior can inadvertently shape the client away from getting back on their meal plan or helping them interrupt dangerous binge–purge cycles as soon as possible. If your client calls after an ED behavior, they are reminded of the phone coaching plan and invited to call if they want help at the next meal/snack. If your client calls at the next meal or snack, you would not discuss the previous behavior (this would be discussed at your next scheduled individual session). Instead, you would focus on the present moment and coach your client to use skills for *this* meal/snack. Your client is encouraged to use phone coaching for any ED behavior.

It is important to note that the 24-hour rule for suicide and self-injury remains firmly intact. Clients may still call for help with ED urges at the next meal/snack following a suicide or self-injury event, provided the call is focused solely on moving forward with ED recovery behaviors, not discussing the previous target behavior. However, therapists should be mindful that repeated calls for ED-related coaching immediately following suicide or self-injury can sometimes reinforce symptom use, especially if the environment primarily targets self-harm. In such cases, careful consultation with your team is essential to ensure you are upholding DBT principles and that coaching continues to shape effective behaviors rather than inadvertently reinforcing life-threatening ones.

## Making It Work

Effectiveness flows from collaborative orientation. When you and your client are on the same page about what phone coaching is, is not, and how to use it, you are more likely to experience phone coaching as beneficial. In addition to the NM/S rule, we orient our clients to the following points before offering any between-session support (keep in mind that phone coaching does not begin until the pretreatment phase is complete and the comprehensive program has started):

- *Phone coaching is a helpful and necessary part of treatment.* Talk with your client about why phone coaching is considered one of the four modes of treatment and how it is structured. It is particularly important to highlight how this treatment component will help them build a life worth living. Discuss the importance of between-session contact and how you will target overuse and nonuse of this aspect of the therapy.
- *Phone coaching is not therapy.* The goal of between-session contact is to help your client access skills. If your client is calling to talk about changing the treatment plan or quitting therapy, you can offer skills to help them cope in that moment until they get to the next scheduled session, but you cannot solve such an important issue on a brief call. We tell our clients that it would be incredibly invalidating if we attempted to do that on a 10-minute phone call! It is important to remind clients that phone coaching is brief. Metaphorically speaking, it acts like a touchstone; a reliable reference point from which to assess something more

stable and grounding. It is like calling your wise mind to determine effective next steps.

- *Phone coaching is not a crisis line.* Dialectically, while we can help our clients during a crisis, we are also not a hospital emergency room or an on-call crisis service. If your client calls for coaching, provide a window of time in which you are likely to respond (e.g., 3 hours). During that time, your client is expected to use their DBT skills to manage until you can speak with them or access crisis services (e.g., emergency room, crisis lines) if they cannot wait.
- *Have a plan for what skills will be used before calling/when waiting for a response.* Coping ahead is essential. We find it helpful to use a skills coaching action plan, filled out ahead of time, that outlines what strategies your client is willing to try before calling for coaching and while waiting for you to respond to their request for support. We work with clients to select skills that would be helpful for the ED behavior they are working on and rehearse their use in session as needed. If, for example, your client is trying to cope with distressing body image, they might use the Wise Mind ACCEPTS skill as follows:
    - ☐ Activities—sit in child's pose for 5 minutes
    - ☐ Comparisons—name three things you are grateful for
    - ☐ Contributing—do some helpful family chores around this house
    - ☐ Emotion—watch 4 minutes of your favorite comedy to generate a different emotion
    - ☐ Push Away—imagine putting your body image distress on a sailboat and watching it float far off into the distance
    - ☐ Thoughts—soften the harsh self-critic by practicing non-judgment toward your body
    - ☐ Sensations—put a heated bean bag on the part of your body that is causing distress
- *Call* ***before*** *acting on urges.* As noted, the aim of phone coaching is to interrupt patterns that lead to symptoms. If your client is trying to stop binge eating, we want them to call as soon as they notice thoughts of planning the binge or as they are driving to the grocery store so we can help link to skills. If they call after binge eating, we can't be helpful! When a client contacts us to say that they have engaged in ED behaviors and they are new to this process, respond by reminding them that

the goal is to address the behavior before it occurs, then end the call and address it as a T2 in the next session):

*Client: I've just binged and purged again, and I was hoping we could talk.*

*Therapist*: Hang on, just to clarify: you have already engaged in the behavior?

*Client*: Yes, I was really stressed and ate some pizza and then it just went from there.

*Therapist*: Got it. I am going to remind you that the goal is to get you to call *before* the behavior. We will need to end the call now, but please know that if you can call me *before* you engage in the behavior, even at the *next* meal or snack, I will have a much better chance of helping you do something different (which I really want to do).

Sometimes, we are asked if clients can call between a binge and a purge (even though these are connected and happen close to one another) or between binge/purge cycles (in cases where a client will engage in several binge/purge episodes back-to-back) to break the cycle. We remind clinicians (and clients) that MED-DBT is principle-driven, not protocol-driven. Yes, there are guidelines around when and how to respond to a client, *and* each circumstance is different. If your efforts to target the binge eating aren't working and purging is causing T1 symptoms (e.g., hypokalemia), this could be a helpful harm reduction strategy.

- *Call with a willingness/openness to problem-solve*. This can be a challenge as clients often tell us that they don't call because they know we are going to ask them to use skills to complete a meal or refrain from purging. We know that eating foods or stopping a binge-purge cycle can feel nearly impossible, and it is possible, but we need some openness to trying something different as shown in the following example.

*Client: I am calling because you told me to call you when I plan to restrict.*

*Therapist*: I *did* ask you to call me when you plan to restrict, so thank you for that. Are you calling because you want to figure out how to eat lunch?

*Client*: Nope.

*Therapist*: Oh, okay. Kinda bummed to hear that.

*Client*: All you want to talk about is eating.

*Therapist*: Yes, at this moment because we agreed to work on increasing food intake to offset the low heart rate.

*Client*: (*silent*)

*Therapist*: . . . and I am not here to force you to eat. I am here if you want my help to figure out how to change that behavior because I know your goal was to stay out of the hospital *and* it is up to you.

*Client*: Well, I can try to eat something, but probably not my whole lunch.

*Therapist*: I can work with that.

*Client*: Okay, fine.

*Therapist*: Great. What skills have you already tried?

- *Get clear on the need.* As in any DBT coaching, helping your clients get clear on what they would like help with usually takes some time in and out of sessions. You may find yourself in the middle of a coaching call trying to solve several problems and wondering if any of it is what the client actually needs help with. The following text message exchange with a client demonstrates how to extinguish value messages and shape more effective coaching requests. This also serves to help our clients become more direct and accurate communicators in general.

*Client: I hate Christmas!*

*Therapist*: Is this an FYI text, or are you wanting my help with something?

*Client*: There are too many family plans and meals, and everyone is cooking and eating!

*Therapist*: Yes, holidays are definitely hard for these reasons. Is there a need in there that I can help with?

*Client*: I don't want to eat or go to any of these things!

*Therapist*: I want to help, but not sure if you want that?

*Client*: I am just letting you know that I am staying home and not eating!

*Therapist*: Oh (*inserts sad emoji*), I thought you were calling for coaching. Okay, thanks for letting me know, and if you need skills help, you know where to reach me.

While it might be tempting to talk about a few skills and call it a day, our clients often need help initiating or maintaining the skill in a difficult moment.

*Client*: Nothing is working!

*Therapist*: What if we try something together? Would you be willing to do that with me?

*Client*: I guess so.

*Therapist*: Okay, what if we try the paced breathing one together? That was one you picked in our last session, right?

*Client*: Yeah, but I tried that and I still want to binge.

*Therapist*: Okay, let's both use the app and do it together if you are still willing.

*Client*: Yeah, okay, give me a second to open it.

*Therapist*: Awesome, thanks. Why don't you put the volume up so we can both hear it?

(*Client's app starts playing a paced breathing exercise that client and therapist do together for 4 minutes. When the cycle ends. . .*)

*Therapist*: So, what are you noticing right now?

*Client*: I've never done it that long before. I actually feel calmer.

*Therapist*: Any change to the urges to binge?

*Client*: I mean, they are still there, but I feel like I am in slow motion now.

*Therapist*: Okay, so that is a change. Let's come up with a plan for you to use a few other skills and see where that takes you.

Be clear about what will burn you both out. It is reasonable to expect that our clients will need support on how to use skills around meals, snacks, and daily urges. It is also true that therapists will be burnt out if their client is calling for every meal/snack. In pretreatment and as needed over the course of treatment, you will need to have a conversation with your client about the ways phone coaching is not effective. We have also been asked whether it is reasonable to only permit clients to call for some ED symptoms. We do not recommend setting arbitrary rules around which ED behaviors to call for. If you do this as a general approach, you won't know what they need or how their symptoms are presenting. For example, observing what the client needs help with through phone coaching will help you determine if they need a higher level of care or whether their behavior can be shaped. Whenever you are observing ineffectiveness (on your part or the client's), this is put on the agenda as a T2 behavior in the next session.

## Summary

Phone coaching in MED-DBT is as essential as the skills groups, individual MED-DBT therapy, and the consult team. Much of the style and practicalities of between-session contact remain identical to how we apply this mode of treatment in standard DBT. The original approach, however, does require modification to meet the needs of our clients and to be effective in treating them in an outpatient setting. Notably, it is necessary for you to be comfortable and confident in using the NM/S rule and to be open and genuine with your clients about what is working and not working, as you use phone coaching together. While phone coaching helps clients apply skills in real time, shaping behavior more broadly requires a deeper understanding of how consequences influence action. In the next chapter, we turn to contingency management—a core component of MED-DBT that uses learning theory to reinforce effective behavior and reduce therapy-interfering patterns. You'll learn how to apply these principles thoughtfully and ethically to support long-term change in clients with multidiagnostic ED presentations.

# 17

# Contingency Management in MED-DBT

Contingency management (CM) is the intentional use of learning theory to shape behavior. It is an important part of MED-DBT, but how it gets used can make or break progress. While using contingencies in the context of therapy may seem straightforward on the outset (if *x*, then *y*), the manner in which your client is oriented to them, how contingencies are chosen, and the way they are applied is complex and nuanced, especially when applied to those living with EDs. In this chapter, we focus on the things you will need to consider in your use of CM in the MED-DBT model.

## What Is CM?

CM is based on operant and classical conditioning principles and is sometimes referred to as motivational or reward incentive planning. As a science, behaviorism is concerned with the manner in which learning is influenced by the environment through systems of conditioning, consequences, and contingencies. We know that the likelihood of a behavior being repeated is directly related to what follows that behavior. For instance, if people laugh at my jokes, then I will tell jokes more often; however, if my jokes are followed by silence then I am less likely to tell jokes! Contingencies themselves are not unique to therapy. All behavior is influenced and shaped by planned and unplanned contingencies. Most of your daily decisions are a result of shaping (e.g., wearing seatbelts to avoid being hurt or accruing a fine, not yelling at your boss in order to keep your job, brushing your teeth after dinner because it gives you a clean feeling). From a behavioral lens, much behavior is learned and can be unlearned (see Linehan, 1993; Swenson,

2016; Koerner, 2011). CM highlights and makes use of the "if–then" relationship between variables.

In the MED-DBT context, CM focuses on helping patients change deeply rooted behaviors through a highly collaborative process in which desired or effective actions are rewarded and maladaptive ones are extinguished. As you read through this chapter, keep in mind that CM is not applied as a stand-alone intervention, but rather in conjunction with the other DBT strategies and assumptions (e.g., dialectics, validation strategies, assumptions about clients). To apply CM without the full DBT philosophy increases the likelihood of it being experienced as punitive and unilateral. It is also important to note that it is not applied to a client: It is a collaborative process whereby we teach clients to change their own behavior.

## Why CM for the Treatment of EDs?

Contingencies are not new to ED treatment. Your clients will know this, and some may feel anxious about this part of MED-DBT depending on their past ED treatment experiences. In higher levels of care, unit privileges and outings may be withheld when patients have not completed a meal. In other contexts, therapists may be unwilling to see a patient at a particular weight or tell them they must go to a higher level of care if their symptoms reach a certain frequency. Of note, some of our clients tell us that they have experienced traditional use of CM as punishing, noncollaborative, and sometimes unhelpful. On the other hand, DBT clinicians are familiar with CM but tend to struggle with how to use them in response to ED behaviors.

The factors that cause and maintain EDs are complex and involve a number of internal and external reinforcers. ED behaviors do not happen arbitrarily, and by the time our clients get to us, those behaviors have been reinforced by the patient, their biology, the environment, and the culture for many years. When they purge, they may feel physical and emotional relief. When they lose weight, people may respond differently to them. When they are medically unstable, they may get admitted to the hospital. When they skip meals, people may make comments about how they admire their willpower. When they overexercise, others may celebrate their commitment to sport. From a neurobiological level, ED behaviors can subdue intolerable body sensations, minimize intense emotions, and calm physiological distress. As a result, behavior change is unlikely to happen without modifying the very powerful factors that reinforce and maintain them. Therefore, MED-DBT pays close attention to the way ED behaviors (alongside other targeted behaviors) arise and are reinforced, using this data to steer the treatment toward life worth living goals. A few points as you get started:

- Everybody and every *body* is different. It is impossible to create a list of all ED-related contingencies or come up with examples that will apply to all clients. It is important not to make assumptions about what causes a behavior to happen repeatedly and instead explore with your clients how their behaviors are reinforced. What is reinforcing for one person (e.g., praise) may be punishing to another person with a different biology and learning history.
- The consequences of a behavior are not the same as the intention of the behavior. Your client might restrict food intake to lose weight and then receive praise from family or healthcare professionals and feel a sense of inclusion and connection they weren't expecting. That connection can become reinforcing. Or your client may purge to get rid of calories and then learn that it makes them feel calm afterward, which can become reinforcing. If we don't separate intent from consequences, we may inadvertently set up ineffective contingencies by overly focusing on variables that are less potent.
- Stay mindful of the way in which your own beliefs and assumptions about body weight, shape, and eating can reinforce your client's behavior. Commenting on weight loss or showing a bias toward "clean eating" in session are likely to reinforce ED symptoms in your clients. Only attending to weight loss and not attending to weight gain is another example of bias. MED-DBT therapists continually work on weight bias and are cognizant of how their own sociocultural beliefs about weight, food, and health might play out in the CM context.
- CM is a collaborative and empowering process. Creating a space where your client can observe and explore existing contingencies without judgment and learn how to harness the power of CM for their own benefit is a hugely empowering and life-changing skill set. Teaching clients that they have more choices and ways to achieve a different outcome than they realize is also reinforcing in its own right.
- It will be important for you to use GIVE skills (emphasizing the importance of the relationship) as you present and negotiate contingencies with your clients. Standard ED treatments tend to be less collaborative

and more rigid in the way behaviors are approached. In some cases, the communication can feel more like a threat than a shared treatment target (e.g., if you don't finish what is on your plate, you will lose privileges). MED-DBT centers the relationship and uses a gentle, curious, validating, and dialectical stance when discussing contingency plans.

## Setting the Stage for Using CM

In MED-DBT, we do not want our behavioral interventions to feel authoritarian; rather, we strive to use contingencies in a way that is highly collaborative and empowering for our clients. Wisniewski and Ben-Porath (2015) say that "the therapist's job in contingency management is not to require the patient to set a particular contingency for a target behavior; rather, the therapist's goal is to notice with the patient how her choice of contingencies does or/does not lead to the patient's desired outcome." CM emerges from a place of curiosity ("What controls this behavior?") and collaboration ("How can we change the pattern so you get more of what you want?"). We achieve this by orienting (and micro-orienting as needed) our clients to the fact that they are already operating within a system of contingencies that may actually be getting in the way of the life they want. This means empowering your client to see how they can modify their own contingencies for their desired outcomes.

One of the first things you will do with your client is to explore how ED (and co-occurring symptoms) behaviors have been reinforced. We want to increase awareness with respect to the complex and unintentional way behaviors are maintained. We also want to help our clients determine which contingencies help them get closer to a life worth living and which interfere with that vision. In keeping with Linehan's CM procedures checklist (Table 10.2 in Linehan, 1993) we provide a brief example of the early phases of orienting a client to CM protocols during MED-DBT pretreatment (notice the therapist's use of CM strategies throughout the dialogue to influence the outcome).

### Background

Giorgi was in the pretreatment phase (Session 2) when her mother called to tell the team that she had been hospitalized over the weekend due to medical instability and suicidal thoughts. She was admitted for three days and discharged back to her family physician. She attended her next scheduled pretreatment session still wearing the hospital identification bracelet on her wrist because "I'll probably be back in a few days anyway, so what's the point of taking it off?"

*Therapist*: Hey. Glad you were able to keep our session. [Reinforcement of effective behavior] I wasn't sure if you would be out of the hospital right away and was thinking I might miss you. [The therapist expresses sadness through facial expression; shaping ineffective behavior via aversive contingency.]

*Giorgi*: (*Shrugs shoulders, looks away*.) I will probably be back there by the weekend. Keeping my ID bracelet on to speed things up.

*Therapist*: Oh! What makes you say that? Do you have a reservation?! [The MED-DBT therapist is purposely not responding to the client's communication the way others might. It is natural that a clinician or family member might feel anxious or annoyed at a comment like this. The important part is *how* one responds in this context. The therapist uses the MED-DBT framework to help her choose how to respond effectively, rather than emotionally. In this scenario, the therapist adopts a lighter stance emphasizing curiosity and irreverence.]

*Giorgi*: (*Laughs*.) I kinda feel like I should have a reservation! It's just the way it goes I guess. I don't plan to eat so that means I will be sent back to the hospital. Just a matter of time.

*Therapist*: Okay, so you have identified that not eating is what leads to getting hospitalized. This is good to know. It gives us a choice [therapist acknowledges the statement without reinforcing it and maintains a curious stance]. Actually, this might be a good time for us to talk about CM in MED-DBT. I would need you to know about it before making a decision about whether we work together. Are you up for talking about that? [collaborative approach, not assuming client wants to learn about this, helps encourage willingness]

*Giorgi*: Sure. That's fine.

*Therapist*: (*Smiles, offering reinforcement of willingness to talk more*.) Okay. Have you heard of contingency management before?

*Giorgi*: Sort of. Isn't it about consequences or something like that? I remember talking about this in one of my psychology undergrad courses.

*Therapist*: Yeah, contingency management is a process of studying what reinforces, or keeps, a behavior going and leveraging that to get you closer to the life you want. You and I would work together to see how certain symptom patterns show up in your life, decide whether the pattern is effective, and then put in contingencies to get a different outcome.

*Giorgi*: Sounds complicated.

*Therapist*: (*Smiles.*) Not when we do it together! [The therapist maintains a collaborative stance reinforcing idea that working together is beneficial and problems can be solved.] I mean there are already lots of contingencies at play right now in your life. The question is whether they are helping you get to the LWL goals you have been talking with me about.

*Giorgi*: Well, I told you that those LWL dreams are too far off. I will probably be dead before I can even try, or the hospital will just keep me there. Either way they aren't likely to happen.

*Therapist*: I agree that the current circumstances make it difficult, if not impossible, to get the life you wish you had. I have an idea. Would it be okay if we use your hospitalization from the weekend as an example of how contingency management might work if we moved forward in this treatment? [The therapist decides to ignore the comment that the LWL dreams are too far off in an early effort to extinguish the behavior by removing her attention as a possible reinforcer. Instead, the therapist validates that the current contingencies make it hard to achieve an LWL and invites further dialogue.]

*Giorgi*: Sure. If you can change this nightmare around, then you have superpowers.

*Therapist*: (*Smiles.*) I mean, I can be pretty skillful, but I definitely don't have superpowers. [Use of the dialectical strategy of oscillating intensity between omnipotence and impotence] I do think together we could shake things up a bit, though, if you wanted to. [The therapist does not reinforce the notion that only someone with superpowers could change the situation, reinforces working together as a solution.]

## Reinforcing Target-Relevant Adaptive Behaviors

As in standard DBT, you will pay attention to and reinforce target-relevant behaviors as they arise using your knowledge of reinforcement principles (e.g., timing, scheduling of reinforcers). You may find that your client's effective behaviors receive little reinforcement (e.g., eating breakfast, gaining weight), especially in weight-centric, diet culture environments. That said, how you reinforce eating and weight can be challenging. For some, an expression of warmth or praise for sticking to the meal plan is effective; for others, it can be experienced as invalidating and superficial and can result in an increase in the very behavior you are trying to reduce. Your job is to get to know what type of responses are reinforcing, knowing that each client is unique. You might find that communicating respect, admiration for, or receiving extra attention from you works better than cheerleading or direct praise for some people in some circumstances:

- Instead of "that's great that you ate breakfast!" consider, "I really respect your effort to eat breakfast today. That isn't an easy thing to do."
- Instead of "great that you gained weight this week," consider "I admire you for how you approach doing hard things, weight gain being one of those."

Showing interest, curiosity, and energy, both verbally and nonverbally are all ways to reinforce effective client behaviors. Leaning in, smiling, expressing warmth when your client talks about a life worth living goal or mentions an idea about countering diet culture are examples of social signals that can reinforce behavior. Shaping small steps toward a desired behavior is also needed. While it might be tempting to focus on why your client left the dinner table after a few bites, it is also important to reinforce the smaller "wins" such as "I noticed that was the first time in a month that you went into the kitchen for dinner" or "I appreciate you trying to sit with your family like we talked about. You even took a few bites. Those are important actions." Those small steps form the foundation for the change you and your client are seeking; don't underestimate them.

## Inadvertent Reinforcement of Target Behaviors

It may be the case that we inadvertently engage with clients in ways that maintain problem behaviors. For example, we may not hold a limit where a limit needs to be held, or we may not use confrontation or a withdrawal of warmth where it could have been helpful in shaping behavior. It is our experience that when there is a behavior that is not changing, the behavior is being inadvertently reinforced, and unless we identify and address the reinforcement, things are unlikely to improve. Some examples of ways we might reinforce a maladaptive pattern include the following:

- Continuing to provide MED-DBT while your client is admitted to an inpatient unit

- Continuing to see a client when they are not willing to work on T1 behaviors (e.g., not willing to get labs done, not willing to follow a harm reduction protocol)
- Not directly addressing purging in a pregnant client
- Spending considerable time after skills group to problem-solve medical instability, especially when the client was unwilling to discuss this in individual therapy
- Extending session time to accommodate lateness or because your client did not complete the food log section of their diary card
- Not addressing ineffective use of phone coaching around meals/snacks
- Withdrawing attention to meal completion because suicide is brought up in that context
- Commenting positively on your client's weight loss

EDs can elicit many different emotions and beliefs in those who treat them. Fidelity to MED-DBT involves being mindful of the ways we reinforce problematic patterns and bringing them to consult team to explore and correct.

## Aversive Contingencies

### Extinguishing Target-Relevant Maladaptive Behaviors

Later on in treatment, Giorgi and her therapist struggled to stop her purging behavior. Although she said she wanted to stop purging, efforts to reinforce effective behavior (e.g., increasing therapist warmth on days of no purging, celebrating the use of skills to try to circumvent purging, more session time to talk about things Giorgi wanted to discuss when purging was reduced) and teach DBT skills to manage urges did not result in enough progress. The therapist asked Giorgi to write a check to an organization that was against her values. Through their discussion, they both agreed that the therapist would keep the check in her office and, if she purged, the therapist would send the check to the organization. This finally worked.

While reinforcement is the preferred approach to shaping behavior, there will be times when, despite your best efforts, aversive contingencies may be necessary. We can reduce or eliminate target behaviors (those determined by the hierarchy) by removing the reinforcers that maintain their presence and/or pairing a target behavior with an aversive consequence. These interventions rely on your knowledge of extinction schedules, aversive consequences, correction-overcorrection protocols, and differences between punishment and punitiveness. Pairing an unwanted outcome (e.g., sending a check to an organization that goes against your values) with a targeted behavior (e.g., purging) can be a potent way of changing habitual behaviors. Aversive contingencies are not the preferred method of shaping behavior so their use must be well-thought-out and appropriately implemented. We use these contingencies primarily in two circumstances:

1. When the reinforcers are not under the control of the therapist and other stronger reinforcers are not available (e.g., restrictions that reduces gastrointestinal distress, excessive exercise that helps to mute emotions, medical instability that results in acceptance into inpatient treatment, increased purging that elicits care and warmth from others).
2. When a behavior is so treatment-interfering that it completely interferes with any kind of adaptive behavior. For example, a client was so angry regarding any type of ED treatment that sessions were dominated by yelling and criticism, resulting in almost no adaptive behavior for the therapist to reinforce. In this case, the therapist responded by ending sessions within 10 minutes of yelling unless the client was willing to change the style of communication.

## Disapproval, Confrontations, and Withdrawal of Warmth

A client struggled to eat and often felt intense anxiety and disgust during meals. This would commonly result in expressions of hopelessness and urges to self-harm. Together with her therapist, the client observed that treatment providers and sometimes her parents would change the type of food offered (to something perceived as safer to the client) or not hold limits around completing a meal when she expressed urges to self-harm. Even though that was not what prompted the thoughts, the unintended consequence of not having to eat became reinforcing. This had never directly been targeted in previous treatments.

For this client, talking about self-harm during meals elicited anxiety from family and some healthcare providers which, in turn, resulted in the removal of the feared stimulus (the meal) which reduced the self-harm urges and eased the anxiety of the care providers (and the patient). This pattern "works" in the short term by decreasing distress but guarantees more intense self-injurious behavior in the future when faced with the inevitable task of eating. What might confronting this pattern look like? How does the therapist withdraw warmth or communicate disapproval effectively in this situation?

We observe and describe the relationship between self-injury and meal completion without judgment ("I have noticed a dynamic at play when you sit down to eat that I think is keeping your self-harm behavior going and vice versa"). You might withdraw warmth when your client talks about not eating or not trying skills at meals by sitting back (rather than leaning in), adopting a facial expression that conveys concern or frustration, or using self-involving self-disclosure ("When you express self-harm as a way to cope with your meals and are not willing to try the skills we practiced, I notice myself feeling some frustration").

Importantly, the use of disapproval or confrontation is thoughtful and strategic. It is not an emotion-minded response by the therapist. It is an intervention, a deliberate and thought-out choice on the therapist's part, borne out of their understanding of this client and their biosocial formulation, used in an effort to elicit more effective behavior. There cannot be a one-size-fits-all approach. What reinforces or shapes one client will not be the same for another. Communicating frustration may move a client to get their lab work done, or your frustration may be received as a sign that you care, thereby maintaining a lack of collaboration around lab work.

## Correction–Overcorrection

Another type of aversive consequence involves a process in which a person both corrects *and* overcorrects for a behavior. For example, a client went home after a session and reported to her parents that their therapist told them they didn't have to gain weight or recover. This led to numerous angry and anxious phone calls and emails from the parents to the therapist over a 48-hour period. In the following session with the client, the therapist (using irreverent and dialectical strategies) directly addressed the behavior ("What happened that you told your parents I said you didn't have to get better or gain weight!") and expressed the impact on them ("When you tell them things that I did not say, their worry results in many angry emails to me and that really pushes my limits"). The therapist and client came up with a plan to correct (e.g., completing a chain and solution analysis) and overcorrect (e.g., the client would give a presentation to her parents outlining what MED-DBT is, how the target hierarchy addresses ED symptoms, and what it means to pursue a life worth living). That was the last time the parents called and the client was more mindful of how she summarized treatment to her family.

In delivering this protocol, you will need to orient your client to it ahead of time and follow the three steps outlined by Linehan (1993):

1. The therapist adds an aversive contingency when a target behavior occurs (withdraws warmth, communicates "It's not okay that you continue to purge while pregnant.").
2. The client is asked to use a new skill or behavior to correct the effects of the target behavior (client agrees to talk with doctor immediately about stabilizing sodium and potassium levels) and overcorrect for it (patient volunteers to keep all bathroom doors open after meals at home to decrease purging and writes a summary about what purging does to the fetus).
3. Once the correct-overcorrect procedure is complete, the therapist immediately stops the aversive contingency (therapist increases warmth, interest).

## Observing Limits Protocol

All healthy relationships involve observing limits. The same is true in the therapy context. MED-DBT is an intensive treatment for both client and therapist, and it is crucial that both parties can express and respond to one another's limits over the course of treatment. Linehan made a distinction between boundaries, which she felt were concrete or unchanging, and limits, which she conceptualized as fluid constructs that wax and wane over time and circumstances. Your limits today may not be the same as your limits in 3 months. Observing limits in MED-DBT, as in standard DBT, requires you to orient clients to your limits, invite your clients to orient you to their limits, and to address the things that push those limits as they arise. Observing limits is considered to be a preventative act, one that when practiced by client and therapist can enhance the relationship and protect against burnout (for both client and therapist).

If you are coming from an ED treatment background, observing limits in MED-DBT may require letting go of commonly held and more rigid boundaries that define standard ED treatments. For example, we don't have a BMI cutoff to engage with treatment or a weekly weight gain expectation. We don't put limits around co-occurring conditions (e.g., "You have to treat your trauma before we can treat your ED") or around specific food rules (e.g., you have to eat this much in this way and during this period of time). It doesn't mean we don't work on these things; rather, we don't put arbitrary limits around a client.

Those trained in standard DBT may not anticipate the ways ED symptoms can push limits (e.g., multiple daily phone coaching calls for meals and snacks, navigating medical risk, working with someone who is at a low body weight and not gaining weight). Keep in mind that many of our clients have experienced limit-setting in punitive or inconsistent ways. Experiences of being "kicked out" of treatment for being "resistant" or "unmotivated" are common for those we treat. In another vein, many clients describe experiences where the people in their lives oscillated between walking on eggshells/not observing limits and having angry or explosive outbursts "out of the blue." In these ways, our clients have never learned how to observe their own or another's limits.

In MED-DBT, we emphasize transparency and honesty and do not avoid talking about things that push our limits. We model and teach our clients to do the same. Using the phenomenological empathy agreement, we view all behavior through a lens of compassion and do not assume ill intent with one another. Limits in MED-DBT might include letting your client know that you will tolerate slower progress *and* that slow progress might burn you out in time. Another example is communicating that you need them to work on reducing purging while pregnant in order to stay in treatment with you. Limits are commonly discussed in your consult team meetings given that they ebb and flow and that we tend to get more rigid or narrow when under stress. We rely on our team to help us uphold DBT team and client agreements. There will be times when increasing your limits is effective (e.g., accepting more phone coaching calls to help with nourishment during a stressful holiday period) and times when you might tighten your limits in order to shape your client's behavior (e.g., not providing phone coaching during a week when your client misses a skills group). Your team can help you reflect on whether your limits are too narrow versus too loose so you can be most effective with your client.

## Therapy Vacations in MED-DBT

Dina was a 45-year-old woman in our MED-DBT program. She had lived with anorexia and type 1 diabetes for more than two decades and had years of different treatments across levels of care. She also had a substantial trauma history and had recurrent episodes of self-harm and suicide attempts. She also faced financial barriers. About seven weeks into the program, Dina's health worsened. She experienced numerous hypoglycemic episodes that required external intervention. She drove an hour each day to and from the treatment center, and the team was very concerned about her ability to maintain safety on the road. She refused to attend appointments with her diabetic care team and was unwilling to carry glucose supplements with her. She often left her insulin at home while out for the day causing her insulin levels to rise dangerously. At other times she misused insulin to facilitate weight loss, a dangerous practice.

Despite numerous interventions by the team to shape, engage, and support Dina, the team was not effective in establishing change. Dina's therapist talked with her about a higher level of care and seeking case management. Her primary care physician wanted her to go into a day treatment program. Dina was not willing to attend other treatments. She wanted to remain on an outpatient basis and felt that higher levels of care were too triggering from a trauma perspective. Her health continued to interfere with her participation in treatment, and her therapist grew increasingly anxious and frustrated.

The concept of a "therapy vacation" was proposed by Linehan (1993) in situations where a break from treatment might paradoxically motivate a return to treatment and an increase in more effective behavior. It is important to emphasize that MED-DBT discourages unilateral termination while also acknowledging the reality of therapy impasses. Therapy vacations are the ultimate aversive contingency and are a late-stage effort to try to keep your client in the program. As aversive as they are, they are still done in the frame that our clients are doing their best and not trying to "sabotage" treatment. When implementing a therapy vacation, it is necessary to ensure the following:

- Your client is aware of the patterns that have led to the impasse.
- Other CM efforts have been applied with limited/no success.
- Your client is oriented to the purpose and rationale for a therapy vacation.
- There are clearly written behavioral targets that need to be addressed in order for therapy to resume.
- A time frame is established in which your client can address the interfering issues and return to treatment.

The team invited Dina to attend part of their consultation team meeting. Maintaining a dialectical stance, the team reviewed the problems in therapy, the impact it was having on Dina and the team, and discussed how much they cared for and were worried about her. The team explained that they did not feel that they could be effective in treatment unless Dina was actively involved with a diabetic care team. In addition, given her medical, psychological, and financial difficulties, the team requested that she be connected to a community case manager. If she wished to return to the program, these criteria would need to be in place along with a willingness to maintain a weight that supported medical stability and a willingness to work on staying alive.

Dina expressed gratitude for the team's care and efforts but did not agree that she needed to manage her diabetes. She asked to meet with her therapist for supportive work instead. The team radically accepted Dina's position and observed their limits, honoring that multiple things were true. Dina did not want to work on treating diabetes, and her therapist was not comfortable offering supportive therapy given the severity of her symptoms. Dina was placed on a therapy vacation with a six-week time frame, and given referrals for supportive counselors. She expressed anger at the team, which made holding this limit challenging. During the first week, Dina left three voice messages with her therapist and two with reception expressing suicidal ideation. Her therapist contacted emergency services each time but did not engage with Dina so as not to reinforce suicidal communication, which was a significant part of this client's history.

Two more weeks passed without any contact from Dina. During the third week, Dina forwarded an email to her individual therapist in which an appointment with the diabetes care team had been scheduled. The team sent back an encouraging email to reinforce this behavior. Dina asked if she could resume sessions with her therapist. Using their GIVE skills, the team emailed Dina both to reinforce that she was trying and to observe that all of the criteria would need to be met in order to resume MED-DBT. Eventually, at the six-week mark, Dina completed the tasks that the team asked of her, and she was able to schedule a meeting with her therapist to discuss next steps in MED-DBT.

## Summary

Using learning theory and applying CM strategies are essential and dynamic aspects of this treatment. Your overall goal is to teach your client to evaluate the usefulness of the existing contingencies in their lives and to modify them or set new contingencies that will help them build the lives they want. Reinforcement is the preferred method, and there will be times when aversive contingencies will be needed. Of course, applying CM effectively, like all components of MED-DBT, requires ongoing reflection, collaboration, and support. In the next chapter, we explore the structure and purpose of the MED-DBT consultation team, a critical space where clinicians receive validation, reduce burnout, maintain treatment fidelity, and problem-solve challenges that arise in complex, high-stakes cases.

# 18

# Consult Teams in MED-DBT

Just as in standard comprehensive DBT, the MED-DBT protocol requires clinicians to attend a weekly consultation team meeting that is consistent with the guidelines and structure set out by Sayrs and Linehan (2019). This chapter outlines the things to consider when running a consult team in MED-DBT.

## Why a Consult Team?

Any comprehensive DBT treatment includes a consultation team meeting (Linehan, 1993). Alongside individual therapy, skills training, and phone coaching, the consultation team meeting is an essential component of the therapy and integral to its success. Clinicians treating multidiagnostic or long-standing EDs have reported higher burnout, greater frustration toward clients and treatment, decreased motivation, and problems with communication and treatment planning (Bommen et al., 2023; Couturier et al., 2021; Marino et al., 2020). While rounding on patients (sharing medical and clinical information about the patient with the team: see the next section) is common practice in ED care, it does not address treatment adherence nor does it support clinicians in managing and overcoming their own challenges with clients. Given that treatment fidelity has been shown to improve therapy outcomes in both DBT and in EDs, we feel it is essential that there is a regular space for practitioners to observe and problem-solve therapy drift.

In our experience, consultation team meetings in MED-DBT are associated with the following:

- Clinicians feeling less burnt out, more supported, and more motivated to work with our clients
- Decreased (unresolved) team polarization
- Greater staff retention and a sense of community
- Clinicians feeling valued, respected, and able to contribute to the team effectively
- Treatment adherence and more positive patient outcomes
- Positive feedback from patients who value that we practice what we preach

As in standard DBT, the function of the MED-DBT consult team is to do the following:

- Reduce therapist burnout
- Increase therapist willingness and motivation to deliver the treatment
- Ensure treatment adherence

The meaning of these functions and the manner in which we achieve them is described throughout this chapter. It is important that any provider joining a MED-DBT team is aware of and in agreement with these goals and processes before starting.

## Rounding on Patients versus Consult Team

Our colleagues who have worked across levels of ED care are familiar with the procedure of rounding on patients. Usually done weekly, but more frequently in the context of day treatment or inpatient settings, rounding on patients is a process in which clinicians report on client status and clinical progress and symptoms. With respect to ED treatment, the issues addressed in rounds are likely to include body weight, meal compliance, physical health indicators, the status of comorbid psychiatric symptoms, and treatment engagement. The focus of this meeting is almost entirely on the patient.

Therapists who treat ED patients in outpatient practices are less likely to have weekly team meetings or regular consultation support with colleagues and are unlikely to be involved in a rounding process. On the other hand, our DBT-trained colleagues are very familiar with consult team protocols but often struggle to help colleagues manage their reactions and areas of difficulty around ED behaviors. They may also need help understanding how to manage ED symptoms such as those addressed in the typical rounds meetings.

In MED-DBT, both meetings are necessary but have different functions. The consult team emphasizes treatment fidelity, therapist vulnerability, and exploration of what gets in the way for the provider. Importantly, the focus is on the clinician, not the patient. This means that not all patients will be discussed each week; instead, team members will seek consultation in the areas where they struggle. We recommend that you attend both rounds and consult team meetings, as we have observed that if people miss rounds, they tend to bring those issues into consult team.

We have been asked whether a separate MED-DBT consult team is needed if a therapist works in a standard DBT clinic. The answer is not necessarily. As we do with DBT-PE, we don't feel there needs to be a separate consult team just to discuss our clients. That said, there can be more team-interfering behavior if some of your colleagues are not trained in EDs and weight science (the consistency agreement helps here). We have had situations where some team members have asked to excuse themselves when talking about EDs (due to personal triggers). Teams need to decide what is effective rather than "right" in the spirit of maintaining fidelity to the model and serving our clients.

## Not Your Usual Team Meeting: Philosophy and Agreements

A consult team operates very differently from most team meetings in mental healthcare and can be a steep learning curve for those new to the model. That said, we assume you already have foundational knowledge and experience with consultation teams and therefore do not review those treatment elements in detail in this text (see Sayrs & Linehan, 2019 for review). Instead, we wish to focus on special considerations that arise in consult team that are unique to MED-DBT.

### Voluntary Participation

Before creating or joining a consultation team, you will want to familiarize yourself with the function and goals to make sure this is a good fit for you. Being mandated into a consult team usually backfires. Thus, it is important for each team member to enter this space freely, with a full understanding of an agreement with the values and expectations that guide these team meetings. Consult teams are emotion-focused, and the team is expected to use DBT philosophy and strategies with one another (e.g., practicing mindfulness at the start of each meeting, doing a chain analysis on a team member who arrives late, observing judgments a team member makes about a person's body weight). As in standard DBT, the MED-DBT consultation team meeting is prioritized and you are expected to attend on time and participate each week. Attending is part of motivation and commitment for the therapist; if you are not able or willing to be on the consult team, you would not take on a MED-DBT client. This is because we do not believe it is possible to support your client (and yourself) and deliver all aspects of this treatment on your own. In our opinion, your participation in consult team is part of what makes this treatment successful.

## Do We Need Someone on My Team with ED Expertise?

Yes, we believe this is essential. You will need at least one person on your team who has a solid understanding of the medical needs and status of your clients and has confidence with respect to understanding ED-specific physical consequences and nutritional needs as well as familiarity with weight science, treatment approaches, and the range of ED presentations. Your team will need members who are adept and able to address ED behaviors with concrete language. Without this, we find that the tendency is to view our client's behavior through the lens of emotion dysregulation and medical/nutritional pieces are missed. If you absolutely cannot recruit someone with this expertise, we do advise that you and your team receive regular consultation from an external provider.

## The Team Culture

As detailed in Part II of this book, each member of the consult team agrees to uphold DBT assumptions about clients (e.g., they want to improve, they cannot fail treatment) and consult team agreements (e.g., consult-to-the-client, consistency agreement). When teams get polarized about treatment or feel stuck in therapy, the agreements and assumptions are used to provide structure and a flexible framework for moving forward.

The team also needs to be well-versed in the way biases around weight, shape, and notions of health will inevitably show up in conceptualizations and responses to clients. Just as we strive to ensure our approaches and teams are anti-oppressive and gender-affirming, our teams work to counter discriminatory or biased views about body weight and eating practices. We have observed that there is a qualitative difference with respect to the way teams talk about eating and body weight compared to suicide and self-injury. With respect to the former, there tends to be more discomfort, perhaps because there is greater uncertainty and nuance involved in addressing EDs (vs. a firm stance when it comes to targeting suicide and self-injury). The unease can also be related to wanting to avoid discomfort for oneself or for others on the team. Unlike suicide/self-injury, we all have relationships with food, eating, and the body.

There are also unique issues of power and privilege at play both in our relationship with our clients and within our teams when it comes to body shapes, sizes, cultural beauty ideals, and definitions of health and recovery. These dynamics need to be brought to team, which is really tough. It might be hard to bring specific ED behaviors that personally impact the clinician *and* the team needs to be able to "go where angels fear to tread" versus walking on eggshells and not addressing the elephants in the room. Recent research highlights the necessity of explicitly addressing structural inequities, weight stigma, and systemic biases in ED treatment settings, emphasizing that teams must be intentional and proactive in integrating these considerations into their clinical and consultation practices (Downs et al., 2025). This, however, can only be accomplished if the team is actively learning about and integrating knowledge of EDs and weight bias on the team.

## "Therapy for the Therapist" Concept

The consult team is designed to be a safe and accountable space for you to explore and target burnout, well-being, adherence, and challenges as they relate to the administration of the treatment. Your team helps you apply DBT skills and strategies to your own behavior rather than focusing on what the client is doing. When working with our clients, it can be easy to lose focus on the therapist when there are medical complications and more urgency in the client's presentation. We find that, in these circumstances, the focus shifts back to the client and their therapy-interfering behavior than on the therapist and their behavior.

The therapy for the therapist stance in MED-DBT means addressing your own biases or triggers around a client's ED presentation and exploring the things that are getting in the way of the treatment. An example of this is the tendency to refer to an outside dietitian or physician to assess and provide support when ED behaviors arise. In some cases, this can cause communication difficulties and philosophical differences about how to move forward. We have observed teams sometimes backing away from managing the ED (e.g., weight status, medical stability) because someone such as an outside provider is doing it. In MED-DBT, we would observe this pattern and use DBT strategies and skills to help the therapist address the ED and what might be getting in the way of doing so (e.g., anxiety, lack of ED knowledge, triggered by the client's weight loss). A MED-DBT consult team is a significant departure from traditional ED team management, thus it is important to reflect on how a consult team works before beginning this treatment. It is also imperative that potential new team members are sufficiently familiar with consult team norms.

## How to Run Your MED-DBT Consult Team

Now that you have a group of MED-DBT trained clinicians together, you are ready to meet weekly. Your consult team operates as a parallel process to the work you are doing with your client. For example, you will notice how each of the structural elements of the team (as described below) mirrors how individual therapy sessions run and function in such a way so as to hold the team to the same practices and interventions as those we treat.

### Team Roles

Team members take turns occupying different roles on the consult team. A team lead is assigned for the month whose job it is to manage the meeting. Other team members take on the roles of observer and note taker (see Sayrs & Linehan, 2019). It is important that all team members rotate through these roles as they reinforce different skill sets that are necessary in the delivery of MED-DBT.

### The Agenda

Most DBT teams establish an agenda before the consult team meeting. As noted, you will put yourself on the agenda board, targeting areas where you struggle, are not adherent, notice strong emotions, or feel burnt out. You can also put yourself on the board to celebrate your own progress (e.g., letting the team know that you feel more confident in teaching radical acceptance around body weight and genetics). As you would in standard DBT, you might ask for the team's help managing a suicidal crisis, increasing empathy toward a client, or decreasing judgmental thoughts about why a client is engaging in self-injury (Table 18.1).

Each agenda item is ranked in terms of priority to discuss on a scale of 1 to 5, where higher numbers reflect items that are time-sensitive or involve serious risk of harm or treatment dropout (e.g., your client is nearing the 4-miss rule, or you feel very frustrated/burnt out with slow progress in terms of ED symptoms/weight gain). Anything that helps you stay adherent can go on the agenda board. Sayrs and Linehan (2019) outline possible agenda items that include the following:

- A skills deficit (e.g., not knowing how to manage suicidal thinking during a meal, unsure how to use radical acceptance for body distress)
- A lack of knowledge (e.g., not knowing evidence-based strategies for ARFID)
- A life circumstance that is affecting the quality of care (e.g., a therapist is experiencing ED thoughts or other mental health difficulties that is impacting treatment)
- A team member's own emotion (e.g., experiencing intense fear about medical instability with a client is impacting treatment adherence)
- Decreased motivation to follow the manual or otherwise engage with the team (e.g., feeling burned out with a client's ambivalence to gain

**TABLE 18.1 Reframing Agenda Items for MED-DBT Consultation Team Meetings**

| Instead of . . . | Try . . . |
|---|---|
| "My client isn't motivated for recovery and refuses to eat." | "I need help increasing my commitment and brainstorming ways to coach my client through meals more effectively." |
| "They don't want to gain weight." | "I notice I am not being dialectical around the way I am thinking about my client and their weight status. I need the team's help to find a middle ground." |
| "Their mother keeps calling and is very angry that we aren't moving fast enough with weight gain." | "I need validation and strategies to increase my compassion for this parent whom I feel judgmental toward." |
| "My client wants to keep their eating disorder." | "I am frustrated because I am unsure how to increase commitment with my client. Help!" |

Copyright © 2026 Anita Federici and Lucene Wisniewski. Reprinted by permission.

weight, having urges to move to supportive therapy rather than stay with MED-DBT)

- One's own or a team member's behavior that interferes with the team's functioning (e.g., feeling afraid to express your clinical recommendations to medical providers, feeling frustrated by a team member who displays weight-biased views)

## Mindfulness Activity

Consult teams start with a mindful practice, both to increase attention to the meeting and to reinforce the importance of practicing the skills ourselves. It can also be helpful to engage in some team discussion about how a given mindful practice applies to EDs. For example, after the team practices writing words with their nondominant hand, you might reflect on how that applies to eating a meal, body disturbances, or changes in weight.

*Reading a Team Agreement.* Following the mindfulness activity, the team lead reads a team agreement (see Chapter 4) each week as a reminder of the framework we agree to use in MED-DBT.

## BCAs for Lateness

The consult team meeting is incredibly important. In our experience, a poorly run consult team usually results in treatment that is inadequately delivered. Thus, any absence or lateness is seen as a loss for the rest of the team who rely on your support and expertise each week. With curiosity and operating within a phenomenological empathic lens, team members use chain analysis to explore their own lateness or absences (and other team-interfering behaviors). This mirrors what is done in individual therapy and like all things in DBT, we practice what we preach.

## Wellness Check-Ins

As with all DBT treatments, the MED-DBT team is a community of therapists treating a community of clients. Linehan placed great value on talking openly about burnout and empathic strain and viewed the camaraderie among team members as a mechanism to revitalize team members and increase therapist commitment to doing DBT. As such, consult teams are proactive around addressing burnout (Swenson, 2016). Sayrs and Linehan (2019) recommend creating a 1-minute space for each team member to rate their weekly burnout on a scale of 0–5, observe their openness to critical feedback, and provide a short personal update to the team. This is a crucial part of the process. Our ability to receive feedback from others, manage different views and opinions, and monitor/treat our burnout is directly related to our work with clients and families. There are many nuances and differences when it comes to determining how to move forward in the context of an ED. Treating and practicing this on our teams helps us develop and maintain a skill set that is transferable to handling opposing views with our clients.

For example, Clinician A feels strongly that your approach to weight gain is too slow and this is causing harm. Parents of the adult client believe that your focus on self-harm is making things worse at home around eating. Clinician B argues that slower weight gain and focusing on emotion regulation with a harm reduction plan in place is necessary right now. The discussion on your consult team heats up. Clinician A is feeling invalidated and does not agree with the approach. Clinician B becomes defensive and is tearful as she also expresses feeling invalidated. How we handle differences in opinions and needs, especially in the highly personalized landscape of eating and body weight, is hugely important to this work! The aim of checking in each week on your burnout, vulnerability, and ability to receive critical feedback is to help you become more aware of yourself in the space and to increase our ability to manage conflict effectively.

## Moving through the Agenda

The remainder of the consult team is spent working through the agenda. The team observer helps to ensure the team stays on track with agenda items, time, and focus. It is most helpful for the team to use video or audio recordings to highlight specific therapist–client interactions and to role-play in order to facilitate skills learning.

*Wrap up:* Leave a few minutes at the end of the consult team to reflect on how the meeting went and whether your team was effective. Koerner's (personal communication, July 23, 2025) "team's bullseye" is an excellent tool for your team to use to reflect on whether they felt intellectually stimulated, were the colleagues they aspired to be, took risks for personal and team growth, and felt helped during the team meeting.

## Summary

In MED-DBT, the consultation team meeting is an essential treatment component. The main aims are to enhance therapist skills, maintain treatment adherence, and bolster motivation while preventing and treating clinician burnout. Traditional ED rounding on clients is unique and separate from the role and function of your consultation team meetings. It is necessary to have people on your team who are fluent in understanding EDs and weight bias to ensure accurate conceptualizations and to help the team balance the need to address the ED in the context of other co-occurring conditions. If you are unable to recruit this expertise, external consultation is strongly recommended. While the consultation team plays a vital role in sustaining effective treatment throughout the course of MED-DBT, every treatment has a beginning, a middle, and an end. In the final chapter, we explore how to navigate endings and transitions with care, whether you're concluding treatment, shifting focus to new stages, or preparing your client for ongoing work with another provider. Ending well is as essential as starting strong, and this chapter will help you approach that process with clarity, intention, and compassion.

# 19

# Transitions and Ending Well

At the start of MED-DBT, we ask our clients to commit to a minimum of 6 months of treatment. What happens at the end of those first 6 months depends on a number of variables. You and your client may decide to end treatment at that point. You both may decide that another round of MED-DBT treatment would be beneficial. You may decide that a higher level of care is necessary or that your client is out of Stage 1 and ready to move into Stage 2 work (e.g., trauma). It may also be the case that your client would benefit from a transfer to another therapist to focus on a new area that you may not be trained in (e.g., cognitive processing therapy). Given that this treatment has not been studied in randomized controlled trials, we rely on recommendations and protocols from the standard DBT literature to guide our philosophy on endings and transitions. In this final chapter, we aim to highlight factors to consider at the end of your initial 6-month commitment.

It is important to remind ourselves that ending well starts way back at the beginning of treatment. Linehan (1993) recommends that therapists talk about the fact that therapy will end at the first session. Certainly, when we orient and gain a collaborative agreement to work together for 6 months, we are acknowledging that there is a beginning and an end to the work we will do together. When we plan for graduations and celebrate the graduation of other clients in skills groups along the way, we model transitioning out of MED-DBT. We talk about, plan for, and develop cope ahead plans for when and how therapy will end. We talk about what will inevitably get in the way of ending well, and we work together to address those challenges. Endings and transitions are natural parts of life and learning to cope effectively with them is part of building lives worth living.

If done well, there are no surprises. In fact, it is a helpful exercise in the beginning to have your client write down how they will know that treatment is working. Endings, like the whole of MED-DBT, are collaborative and co-constructed. They are another skillful step in your client's journey and important in terms of helping them continue to build their support networks (versus only relying solely on you to help them). Therapy endings are deeply meaningful rites of passage for you and your client. As Linehan wrote, "DBT does not advocate for a complete rupture in the relationship; instead, the patient moves from the category of patient to that of ex-patient" (1993, p. 457), similar to that of student versus ex-student. As we do in standard DBT, we reinforce self-reliance as well as the need to depend on others for support, we evaluate progress regularly and collaboratively, and we clarify how our relationship with our client will change after MED-DBT ends. So, when do you actually end?!

## Deciding to End or Continue Treatment after the First 6 Months

While we find that most of our clients benefit from a year of MED-DBT, a 6-month dose can be enough to calm the behavioral dyscontrol of Stage 1 for some clients. As you will recall, Stage 1 is characterized by extreme behavioral difficulties that include life-threatening and therapy-interfering behaviors. Moving on from Stage 1 means that your client is able to manage emotions, food, and weight without lapsing into medical instability or relying on frequent ED behaviors, suicide, or self-injury to cope. It also means that you and your client have successfully eliminated (or drastically reduced) treatment-interfering behavior.

In this situation, and depending on the needs of your client, you could end at the 6-month point. It may also be the case, particularly in the fee-for-service context, that your client can only afford a 6-month protocol and has no choice but to end. It is important to emphasize that we don't really expect that people are "cured" at the end of 6 months. These are individuals who present with significant behavioral and emotional issues, and getting them under control is a great step. At the end of this, they may choose to take a break or be able to benefit and tolerate more traditional therapies.

For other clients, 6 months of MED-DBT is not enough of a dose, and you and your client may decide that a second round of treatment would be beneficial. Clients in MED-DBT are able to renew their treatment agreement at the end of 6 months if progress is being made and clear goals are established that will define the next round of care. It is important to address how challenges in the first 6 months will be addressed differently in the second round of treatment so as not to repeat dynamics that hindered progress (for both the therapist and the client). Overall, we want MED-DBT to be successful. Renewing the agreement signifies that there is enough momentum and change happening to support the usefulness of the treatment but that more time and/or new strategies are needed to tackle remaining Stage 1 behaviors.

## Deciding That a Higher Level of Care Is Necessary

Sometimes, in spite of our best efforts, your client will need more than outpatient care. While this may come up before the 6-month mark, it is crucial for you and your client to identify whether stepping up to a higher level of care may be helpful. In one of our programs, we have the benefit of MED-DBT across levels of care (e.g., outpatient, partial hospitalization, and day treatment). In this way, our clients can step up or down in level of intensity but remain in the MED-DBT framework. We recognize this is not the case in many settings. In the latter circumstance, as the 6 months start to come to a close, you and your client will review whether continuing on an outpatient basis makes sense or whether a break from MED-DBT to access a higher level of care would result in greater progress. In this circumstance, you might contract with your client to continue to see them for three to four sessions while they wait to get into care. For example, we negotiated with one client that we would see her weekly while she waited the six weeks for a spot to open up in day treatment as long as she saw her physician weekly to monitor medical stability. These interim sessions focused solely on helping the client get ready for day treatment (e.g., developing cope ahead plans for experiences she feared on the unit like eating feared foods and being weighed).

## Starting Stage 2 Work with You or Another Therapist

Stage 2 focuses on treating PTSD and other trauma-related symptoms, including traumatic invalidation—work that could not have been done earlier due to the severe nature of your client's Stage 1 behaviors. We view Stage 1 MED-DBT as early, foundational trauma work in which our clients learn to manage intense emotions, thoughts, and urges without the ED or other destructive behavior. As Harned (2022) describes in her DBT-PE protocol, while many of our clients are motivated to work on trauma early on, our experience is that they are not able to do so without greater scaffolding around them. Going into exposure work or starting other evidence-based trauma protocols too soon for our clients tends to exacerbate other symptoms (e.g., increase in suicidality, restriction, purging). If, after 6 months of treatment your client demonstrates an ability to consistently manage Stage 1 behaviors, they may be ready to tolerate traditional trauma treatments. This may mean staying with you to do trauma work (e.g., cognitive processing therapy, prolonged exposure, eye movement desensitization and reprocessing) or transitioning to a new therapist with that expertise. It is very important, however, that there is continued awareness of the ED (and other Stage 1 targets) as you move forward. ED behaviors can return quickly and it is important that you and your client remain vigilant to subtle urges or behaviors and continue to practice with relapse prevention at the forefront. It can be tempting to feel like "all of that is behind you" as you move into Stage 2 work, and we have to remember that EDs are neurobiological in nature with periods of relapse and remission. Continued awareness of the ED is part of Stage 2 work and you will need to be able to flexibly shift back to Stage 1 treatment when needed.

For other clients, working on Stage 3 goals (e.g., ordinary problems in living) may be the next step. This might involve a concentrated focus on OCD, body image, mindfulness-based stress reduction to cope with chronic pain, or other areas of difficulty that cause problems with respect to quality of life.

A note on tapering down and booster sessions: Abrupt endings are not advised. The use of a tapering schedule is preferred where your client can begin to practice managing outside of the MED-DBT team context in a gradual fashion. This may mean moving to biweekly sessions and fading out phone coaching in a manner that will encourage skill generalization. Booster sessions may be planned for and scheduled (e.g., every three or 6 months). We emphasize to our clients that they can always return to treatment should the need arise. While the nature of post-MED-DBT contact will vary based on client and therapist circumstances, it should be clearly defined. Joining MED-DBT grad groups is another option for our clients.

## Common Obstacles

### An Increase in Life-Threatening Behaviors

Endings produce powerful emotions and can stir up old ways of coping. The MED-DBT therapist–client relationship is a powerful one, and graduating, while an important accomplishment, usually means moving on to another provider, enrolling in a graduate group, or taking a break from treatment. For some clients, a regression in symptoms may arise during this phase of treatment.

Dylan, a 28-year-old cisgender male client, had been doing very well and was approaching the end of his eleventh month in MED-DBT (he had chosen to do two rounds of MED-DBT for a total of 1 treatment year). He had not engaged in any self-harm behavior for 6 months and had just passed 3 months without any ED behaviors. Dylan and his therapist had a graduation celebration planned, and Dylan had a strong relapse prevention plan in place. As the last four weeks of treatment came to a close, Dylan experienced a rapid return of cutting and daily purging that resulted in an admission to the emergency room. The team was polarized in terms of what to do: Several recommended extending treatment to support Dylan while others felt strongly that ending at the agreed upon graduation date was necessary.

Knowing precisely when to end, especially in the context of medical urgency, can be challenging to discern. There is no single correct response in situations like this. DBT is a principle-driven treatment, and decisions must be guided by a careful exploration of the client's behavior, the function of symptoms, and the principles of the treatment model. We encourage teams to collaboratively assess situations like Dylan's using the following considerations:

- Have you adequately addressed treatment ending over the course of treatment (i.e., is your client prepared and able to end)?
- What function might the return of symptoms serve?
- Is the client showing signs of a behavioral burst?
- What does your client wish to do/what are their suggestions in terms of ending or not?
- If treatment is extended, what contingencies (intended or unintended) might be reinforced?
- What are the pros and cons of holding to, or shifting, the original end date?
- Has the team fully consulted with each other or with outside MED-DBT experts to gain clarity?

In Dylan's case, the team decided, after much discussion, to extend treatment by four additional weeks. This choice was made in close collaboration with Dylan, who expressed a clear desire to understand what had triggered his relapse and to reestablish stability before ending. The final four sessions were used to revisit relapse prevention strategies and solidify his confidence in using skills. Dylan regained stability, and graduation took place the following month, providing a sense of closure and achievement.

This is *one example* of how a team may choose to proceed, but it is not the only valid path. Another approach might be to observe the treatment boundary and hold the original end date, communicating compassion and belief in Dylan's capacity to use skills and his crisis plan, while offering a booster session two weeks later to check in on stability and reinforce treatment gains. In some cases, a client may choose to re-engage in a new round of MED-DBT after a planned break or transition into a different type of care.

When teams find themselves polarized, this is not uncommon, *and* it is essential to continue the conversation until a coherent, principle-aligned course of action emerges. DBT principles, such as balancing acceptance and change, and DBT assumptions about clients, must remain central to these discussions. Treatment endings are as meaningful as treatment beginnings. The clarity, consistency, and intentionality with which endings are handled can have lasting impact on a client's confidence in themselves and their recovery path.

## Summary

It is a wonderful accomplishment to complete treatment, whether that is 6 months or more. The journey into and through MED-DBT takes much willingness, trust, and practice. Celebrating the achievements of our clients and continuing to communicate our belief in their capacity to build lives worth living is at the heart of the model. As we have outlined in this chapter and throughout this book, the seeds for successful treatment transitions are planted very early in treatment. Decision making around when to end treatment and when to transition into another type of treatment is meant to be a collaborative and iterative process. As you move forward in your work with clients, we hope this book has offered both practical guidance and a renewed sense of purpose. MED-DBT is not just a treatment model, it is a compassionate, flexible, and deeply respectful approach to helping individuals navigate some of the most complex and painful experiences of their lives. Thank you for joining us in this work. We are glad you're here.

# List of Abbreviations

| | |
|---|---|
| 2SLGBTQ+: | Two-Spirit, lesbian, gay, bisexual, transgender, queer or questioning |
| AAN: | atypical anorexia nervosa |
| AFT: | adolescent-focused therapy |
| AIWS: | Alice in Wonderland Syndrome |
| AN: | anorexia nervosa |
| AN-B/P: | anorexia nervosa binge–purge subtype |
| AN-R: | anorexia nervosa restricting subtype |
| ARFID: | avoidant–restrictive food intake disorder |
| ASD: | autism spectrum disorder |
| BCA: | behavior-chain analysis |
| BED: | binge-eating disorder |
| BMI: | body mass index |
| BN: | bulimia nervosa |
| BPD: | borderline personality disorder |
| BT: | behavior therapy |
| CBT: | cognitive-behavioral therapy |
| CBT-E: | enhanced cognitive-behavioral therapy |
| CBT-ED: | CBT for eating disorders |
| CM: | contingency management |
| CPT: | cognitive processing therapy |
| DBT-BED: | DBT skills training for binge-eating disorder |

DBT-BN: DBT skills training for bulimia
DBT-PE: dialectical behavior therapy—prolonged exposure
DBT-SUD: dialectical behavior therapy for substance use disorder
DT: distress tolerance
EBT: evidence-based treatment
ED: eating disorder
EMDR: eye movement desensitization and reprocessing
FBT: family-based treatment
HLOC: higher level of care
IPT: interpersonal therapy
LOC: level of care
LWL: life worth living
MLA: missing links analysis
NM/S: next meal/snack rule
NSSI: nonsuicidal self-injury
OCD: obsessive–compulsive disorder
OCPD: obsessive–compulsive personality disorder
OSFED: other specified feeding/eating disorder
PE: prolonged exposure
PTSD: posttraumatic stress disorder
RCT: randomized controlled trial
RD: registered dietitian
RO-DBT: radically open DBT
SH: self-harm
SI: suicidal ideation
SSCM: supportive clinical management
TIBs: therapy-interfering behaviors

# References


Academy for Eating Disorders. (2021). *Eating disorders: A guide to medical care* (4th ed.). Author.

Academy for Eating Disorders. (2023). *Eating disorders: Critical points for early recognition and medical risk management in the care of individuals with eating disorders* (4th ed.). Author.

Alberga, A. S., Russell-Mayhew, S., von Ranson, K. M., & McLaren, L. (2016). Weight bias: A call to action. *Journal of Eating Disorders, 4,* Article 34.

American Psychiatric Association. (2013). Diagnostic and statistical manual of mental disorders (5th ed.). American Psychiatric Publishing.

American Psychiatric Association. (2022). *Diagnostic and statistical manual of mental disorders* (5th ed., text rev.). Author.

American Psychiatric Association. (2023). *Practice guideline for the treatment of patients with eating disorders.* American Psychiatric Publishing.

Anderson, K., Watters, A., Dee, E., & Mehler, P. S. (2023). Can we predict the development of acute gastric dilatation in patients with anorexia nervosa? *Journal of Eating Disorders, 11,* Article 212.

Antuña-Camblor, C., Gómez-Salas, F. J., Burgos-Julián, F. A., González-Vázquez, A., Juarros-Basterretxea, J., & Rodríguez-Díaz, F. J. (2024). Emotional regulation as a transdiagnostic process of emotional disorders in therapy: A systematic review and meta-analysis. *Clinical Psychology & Psychotherapy, 31*(3), e2997.

Arcelus, J., Mitchell, A. J., Wales, J., & Nielsen, S. (2011). Mortality rates in patients with anorexia nervosa and other eating disorders: A meta-analysis of 36 studies. *Archives of General Psychiatry, 68*(7), 724–731.

Asaria, A. (2023). 'Terminal anorexia': A lived experience perspective on the proposed criteria. *Journal of Eating Disorders, 11,* 222.

Asaria, A. (2025). Improving eating disorder care for underserved groups: A lived experience and quality improvement perspective. *Journal of Eating Disorders, 13,* Article 11.

Astrachan-Fletcher, E., & Maslar, M. (2009). *The dialectical behavior therapy skills workbook for bulimia: Using DBT to break the cycle and regain control of your life.* New Harbinger Publications.

Attia, E., & Walsh, B. T. (2025). Eating disorders: A review. *JAMA, 333*(14),1242–1252.

Bankoff, S. M., Karpel, M. G., Forbes, H. E., & Pantalone, D. W. (2012). A systematic review of dialectical behavior therapy for the treatment of eating disorders. *Eating Disorders, 20*(3), 196–215.

Baudinet, J., Simic, M., Griffiths, H., Donnelly, C., Stewart, C., & Goddard, E. (2020). Targeting maladaptive overcontrol with radically open dialectical behaviour therapy in a day programme for adolescents with restrictive eating disorders: An uncontrolled case series. *Journal of Eating Disorders, 8*(1), 68.

Becker, K. R., Mancuso, C., Dreier, M. J., Asanza, E., Breithaupt, L., Slattery, M., et al. (2021). Ghrelin and PYY in low-weight females with avoidant/restrictive food intake disorder compared to anorexia nervosa and healthy controls. *Psychoneuroendocrinology, 129,* 105243.

Ben-Porath, D., Duthu, F., Luo, T., Gonidakis, F., Compte, E. J., & Wisniewski, L. (2020). Dialectical behavioral therapy: An update and review of the existing treatment models adapted for adults with eating disorders. *Eating Disorders, 28*(2), 101–121.

Ben-Porath, D. D., Wisniewski, L., & Warren, M. (2009). Differential treatment response for eating disordered patients with and without a comorbid borderline personality diagnosis using a dialectical behavior therapy (DBT)-informed approach. *Eating Disorders, 17,* 225–241.

Ben-Porath, D. D., Federici, A., Wisniewski, L., & Warren, M. (2014). Dialectical behavior therapy: Does it bring about improvements in affect regulation in individuals with eating disorders? *Journal of Contemporary Psychotherapy, 44*(4), 245–251.

Bhatnagar, K. C., Martin-Wagar, C. A., & Wisniewski, L. (2017). DBT for eating disorders: An overview. In M. Swales (Ed.), *Oxford handbook of dialectical behaviour therapy* (pp. 573–594). Oxford University Press.

Bommen, D., Smith, J., & Lee, A. (2023). 'Helper' or 'punisher'? A qualitative study exploring staff experiences of treating severe and complex eating disorder presentations in inpatient settings. *Journal of Eating Disorders, 11*(1), Article 216.

Brizzi, G., Sansoni, M., Di Lernia, D., Frisone, F., Tuena, C., & Riva, G. (2023). The multisensory mind: A systematic review of multisensory integration processing in Anorexia and Bulimia Nervosa. *Journal of Eating Disorders, 11*(1), 204.

Brown, A., McClelland, J., Hodsoll, J., Lang, K., Boysen, E., Flynn, M., et al. (2019a). A pilot evaluation of a novel First Episode and Rapid Early Intervention service for Eating Disorders (FREED). *European Eating Disorders Review, 27*(1), 55–64.

Brown, A., McClelland, J., Hodsoll, J., Lang, K., Boysen, E., Flynn, M., et al. (2019b). The effectiveness of a novel First Episode and Rapid Early Intervention service for Eating Disorders (FREED): A pilot randomized controlled trial. *European Eating Disorders Review, 27(1)*, 65–74.

Brown, T. A., Cusack, A., Anderson, L. K., Trim, J., Nakamura, T., Trunko, M. E., & Kaye, W. H. (2018). Efficacy of a partial hospital programme for adults with eating disorders. *European Eating Disorders Review, 26*(3), 241–252.

Bulik, C. M. (2005). Exploring the gene–environment nexus in eating disorders. *Journal of Psychiatry & Neuroscience, 30*(5), 335–339.

Bulik, C. M. (2024). Building confidence in discussing genetics with patients with eating disorders and their families. *Focus, 22*(3), 322–327.

Bulik, C. M., Blake, L., & Austin, J. (2019). Genetics of eating disorders: What the clinician needs to know. *Psychiatric Clinics of North America, 42*(1), 59–73.

Bulik, C. M., Flatt, R., Abbaspour, A., & Carroll, I. (2019). Reconceptualizing anorexia nervosa. *Psychiatry and Clinical Neurosciences, 73*(9), 518–525.

Bulik, C. M., Carroll, I. M., & Mehler, P. (2021). Reframing anorexia nervosa as a metabo-psychiatric disorder. *Nature Reviews Drug Discovery, 23*(4), 261–262.

Bulik, C. M., Carroll, I., Mehler, P. S., & Reichborn-Kjennerud, T. (2021). Reframing anorexia nervosa as a metabo-psychiatric disorder. Trends in Endocrinology & Metabolism, 32(10), 752–761.

Bulik, C. M., Berkman, N. D., Brownley, K. A., Sedway, J. A., & Lohr, K. N. (2007). Anorexia nervosa treatment: A systematic review of randomized controlled trials. *International Journal of Eating Disorders, 40*(4), 310–320.

Burke, F., Higgins, M., & MacGinley, M. (2024). "I'll do it on my own, but I'm never alone": Lived experience and practitioner perspectives of autonomy in longstanding and severe eating disorder treatment and recovery–a rapid evidence review. *Journal of Eating Disorders 12*(208), 1–21.

Burke, N. L., Schaefer, L. M., Hazzard, V. M., Rodgers, R. F., & Thompson, J. K. (2020). Where identities converge: The importance of intersectionality in eating disorders research. *International Journal of Eating Disorders*, 53(10), 1605–1609.

Burton Murray, H., Riddle, M., Rao, F., McCann, B., Staller, K., Heitkemper, M., & Kuo, B. (2022). Eating disorder symptoms, including avoidant/restrictive food intake disorder, in patients with disorders of gut–brain interaction. *Neurogastroenterology & Motility, 34*(8), e14258

Carter, J. C., Kenny, T. E., Singleton, C., Van Wijk, M., & Heath, O. (2019). Dialectical behaviour therapy self-help for binge-eating disorder: A randomized controlled study. *International Journal of Eating Disorders, 53*(3), 451–460.

Cerolini, S., Vacca, M., Zegretti, A., Zagaria, A., & Lombardo, C. (2024). Body shaming and internalized weight bias as potential precursors of eating disorders in adolescents. *Frontiers in Psychology, 15*, 1356647.

Chapman, A. L. (2019). *Phone coaching in dialectical behavior therapy*. Guilford Press.

Chapman, A. L., & Rosenthal, M. Z. (2015). *Managing therapy-interfering behavior: Strategies from dialectical behavior therapy*. American Psychological Association

Chen, E. Y., Matthews, L., Allen, C., Kuo, J. R., & Linehan, M. M. (2008). Dialectical behavior therapy for clients with binge-eating disorder or bulimia nervosa and borderline personality disorder. *International Journal of Eating Disorders, 41*(6), 505–512.

Chen, E. Y., Segal, K., Weissman, J., Zeffiro, T. A., Gallop, R., Linehan, M. M., et al. (2015). Adapting dialectical behavioral therapy for adult anorexia nervosa–A pilot study. *International Journal of Eating Disorders, 48*(1), 123–132.

Courbasson, C., Nishikawa, Y., & Dixon, L. (2012). Outcome of dialectical behaviour therapy for concurrent eating and substance use disorders. *Clinical Psychology & Psychotherapy, 19*(5), 434–449.

Couturier, J., Kimber, M., & Szatmari, P. (2013). Efficacy of family-based treatment for adolescents with eating disorders: A systematic review and meta-analysis. *International Journal of Eating Disorders, 46*(1), 3–11.

Couturier, J., Ma, Z., Rahman, L., & Webb, C. (2021). A mixed methods exploratory evaluation of burnout in frontline staff implementing dialectical behavior therapy on a pediatric eating disorders unit. *Journal of Eating Disorders*, 9(98).

Crow, S. J. (2023). Terminal anorexia nervosa cannot currently be identified. *International Journal of Eating Disorders, 56*(7), 1329–1334.

Crowell, S. E., Beauchaine, T. P., & Linehan, M. M. (2009). A biosocial developmental model of borderline personality: Elaborating and extending linehan's theory. *Psychological Bulletin*, 135(3), 495–510.

Czyz, E. K., Berona, J., & King, C. A. (2016). Rehospitalization of suicidal adolescents in relation to course of suicidal ideation and future suicide attempts. *Psychiatric Services (Washington, D.C.), 67*(3), 332–338.

Dalle Grave, R., Sartirana, M., Sermattei, S., & Calugi, S. (2021). Treatment of eating disorders in adults versus adolescents: Similarities and differences. *Clinical Therapeutics, 43*(1), 70–84.

Dansky, B. S., Brewerton, T. D., Kilpatrick, D. G., & O'Neil, P. M. (1997). The National Women's study: Relationship of victimization and posttraumatic stress disorder to bulimia nervosa. *International Journal of Eating Disorders, 21*(3), 213–228.

Day, S., Hay, P., Tannous, W. K., Fatt, S. J., & Mitchison, D. (2024). A systematic review of the effect of PTSD and trauma on treatment outcomes for eating disorders. *Trauma, Violence, & Abuse, 25*(2), 947–964.

DeJong, H., Broadbent, H., & Schmidt, U. (2012). A systematic review of dropout from treatment in outpatients with anorexia nervosa. *The International Journal of Eating Disorders, 45*(5), 635–647.

Deloitte Access Economics. (2020, June). *The social and economic cost of eating disorders in the United States of America: A report for the Strategic Training Initiative for the Prevention of Eating Disorders and the Academy for Eating Disorders*. Author.

Dimeff, L. A., McMain, S., Sayrs, J. H. R., Wilks, C., & Linehan, M. M. (2021). DBT for individuals with borderline personality disorder and substance use disorders. In L. A. Dimeff, S. L. Rizvi, & K. Koerner (Eds.), *Dialectical behavior therapy in clinical practice: Applications across disorders and settings* (2nd ed., pp. 145–173). Guilford Press.

Downs, J. (2021). Finding the middle ground: Building a life worth living with Dialectical Behaviour Therapy. In J. Downs, M. Hopfenbeck, H. Lewis, I. Parker, & N. Schnackenberg (Eds.), *The practical handbook of eating difficulties* (pp. 265–274). Pavilion Publishing and Media Ltd.

Downs, J. (2024a). The body is not just impacted by eating disorders—biology drives them. *Trends in Molecular Medicine, 30*(4), 301–304.

Downs, J. (2024b). Care pathways for longstanding eating disorders must offer paths to recovery, not managed decline. *BJPsych Bulletin, 48*(3), 177–181.

Downs, J., & Mycock, G. (2022). Eating disorders in men: Limited models of diagnosis and treatment are failing patients. *BMJ, 376,* o537.

Downs, J., Adams, J., Federici, A., Sharpe, H., & Ayton, A. (2025). Equity in eating disorders: A dialectical approach to stigma, expertise, and the coproduction of knowledge. *Journal of Eating Disorders, 13*(1), 31.

Downs, J., Ayton, A., Collins, L., Baker, S., Missen, H., & Ibrahim, A. (2023). Untreatable or unable to treat? Creating more effective and accessible treatment for long-standing and severe eating disorders. *The Lancet Psychiatry, 10*(2), 146–154.

Doyle, P. M., & Le Grange, D. (2019). Family-based treatment for adolescent anorexia nervosa: A narrative review. *Journal of Eating Disorders,* 7(1), 6.

Duncan, L., Yilmaz, Z., Gaspar, H., Walters, R., Goldstein, J., Anttila, V., et al. (2017). Significant locus and metabolic genetic correlations revealed in genome-wide association study of anorexia nervosa. *American Journal of Psychiatry, 174*(9), 850–858.

Eddy, K. T., Tabri, N., Thomas, J. J., Murray, H. B., Keshaviah, A., Hastings, E., & Franko, D. L. (2017). Recovery from anorexia nervosa and bulimia nervosa at 22-year follow-up. *Journal of Clinical Psychiatry, 78*(2), 184–189.

Edwards, E. R., Kober, H., Rinne, G. R., Griffin, S. A., Axelrod, S., & Cooney, E. B. (2021). Skills-homework completion and phone coaching as predictors of therapeutic change and outcomes in completers of a DBT intensive outpatient programme. *Psychological Psychotherapy: Theory, Research & Practice, 94*(3), 504–522.

Ejdemyr, I., Sundqvist, R., Bjureberg, J., Birgegård, A., Jokinen, J., Levallius, J., … Sjögren, M. (2025). Feasibility and potential efficacy of radically open dialectical behavior therapy for anorexia nervosa. *Eating Disorders,* 1–19.

Eisler, I., Dare, C., Hodes, M., Russell, G., Dodge, E., & Le Grange, D. (2000). Family therapy for adolescent anorexia nervosa: The results of a controlled comparison of two family interventions. *Journal of Child Psychology and Psychiatry, 41*(6), 727–736.

Eneva, K. T., Murray, S., O'Garro-Moore, J., Yiu, A., Alloy, L. B., Avena, N. M., & Chen, E. Y. (2017). Reward and punishment sensitivity and disordered eating behaviors in men and women. *Journal of Eating Disorders, 5,* Article 6.

Fairburn, C. G. (2008). *Cognitive behavior therapy and eating disorders.* Guilford Press.

Fairburn, C. G., Marcus, M. D., & Wilson, G. T. (1993). Cognitive-behavioral therapy for binge eating and bulimia nervosa: A comprehensive treatment manual. In C. G. Fairburn & G. T. Wilson (Eds.), *Binge eating: Nature, assessment, and treatment* (pp. 361–404). Guilford Press.

Fairburn, C. G., Jones, R., Peveler, R. C., Hope, R. A., & O'Connor, M. (1993). Psychotherapy and bulimia nervosa: Longer-term effects of interpersonal psychotherapy, behavior therapy, and cognitive behavior therapy. *Archives of General Psychiatry, 50*(6), 419–428.

Fairburn, C. G., Jones, R., Peveler, R. C., Hope, R. A., & O'Connor, M. (1995). Psychotherapy and bulimia nervosa: Longer-term effects of interpersonal psychotherapy, behavior therapy, and cognitive behavior therapy. *Archives of General Psychiatry, 52*(4), 337–344.

Favier, M., Martin Garcia, E., Icick, R., de Almeida, C., Jehl, J., Desplanque, M., et al. (2024). The human VGLUT3-pT8I mutation elicits uneven striatal DA signaling, food or drug maladaptive consumption in male mice. *Nature Communications, 15*(1), 5691.

Federici, A., & Kaplan, A. S. (2008), The patient's account of relapse and recovery in anorexia nervosa: A qualitative study. *European Eating Disorders Review, 16,* 1–10.

Federici, A., & Wisniewski, L. (2012). Integrating dialectical behavior therapy and family-based treatment for multidiagnostic adolescent patients. *Journal of Counseling & Development, 90*(3), 330–338.

Federici, A., & Wisniewski, L. (2013). An intensive DBT program for patients with multidiagnostic eating disorder presentations: A case series analysis. *International Journal of Eating Disorders, 46*(4), 322–331.

Federici, A., & Wisniewski, L. (2015). Dialectical behavior therapy for clients with complex and multidiagnostic eating disorder presentations. In L. H. Choate (Ed.), *Eating disorders and obesity: A counselor's guide to prevention and treatment* (pp. 375–398). American Counseling Association.

Federici, A., Wisniewski, L., & Ben-Porath, D. (2012). Description of an intensive dialectical behavior therapy program for multidiagnostic clients with eating disorders. *Journal of Counseling & Developmental, 90,* 330–338.

Friedrich, M. U., Baughan, E. C., Kletenik, I., Younger, E., Zhao, C. W., Howard, C., et al. (2024). Lesions causing Alice in Wonderland syndrome map to a common brain network linking body and size perception. *Annals of Neurology, 96,* 662–674.

Friedrich, M. U., Baughan, E. C., Kletenik, I., Younger, E., Zhao, C. W., Howard, C., Ferguson, M. A., et al. (2024). Lesions causing Alice in Wonderland syndrome map to a common brain network linking body and size perception. Annals of Neurology. Advance online publication.

Fruzzetti, A. E. (2006). *The high conflict couple: A dialectical behavior therapy guide to finding peace, intimacy, and validation.* New Harbinger.

Fruzzetti, A. E., Shenk, C., & Hoffman, P. D. (2005). Family interaction and the development of borderline personality disorder: A transactional model. *Development and Psychopathology, 17*(4), 1005–1027.

Gadsby, S. (2017). Distorted body representations in anorexia nervosa. *Consciousness and Cognition, 51,* 17–33.

Gadsby, S. (2018). How are the spatial characteristics of the body represented? A reply to Pitron & de Vignemont. *Consciousness and Cognition, 62*(February), 163–168.

Galen, G., & Aguirre, B. (2021). *DBT for dummies*. Wiley.

Geller, J., Cockell, S. J., & Goldner, E. M. (2000). Inhibited expression of negative emotions and interpersonal orientation in anorexia nervosa. *International Journal of Eating Disorders, 28*(1), 8–19.

Geller, J., Srikameswaran, S., Zelichowska, J., & Williams, K. D. (2012). Working with severe and enduring eating disorders: Enhancing engagement and matching treatment to client readiness. In J. Fox & K. Goss (Eds.), *Eating and its disorders* (pp. 412–426). Wiley Blackwell. https://doi.org/10.1002/9781118328910.ch26

Giel, K. E., Thiel, A., Teufel, M., Mayer, J., & Zipfel, S. (2010). Weight bias in work settings: A qualitative review. *Obesity Facts, 3*(1), 33–40.

Goldman-Mellor, S. J., Bhat, H. S., Allen, M. H., & Schoenbaum, M. (2022). Suicide risk among hospitalized versus discharged deliberate self-harm patients: Generalized random forest analysis using a large claims data set. *American Journal of Preventive Medicine, 62*(4), 558–566.

Granato, H., Hawkey, C., Kinnear, M., Kleiber, B., Loerinc, A., Murray, A., Rindlaub, L., & Schmidt, S. (2021). Dialectical agreement: We agree to open source anti-discrimination agreements. Synthesis Psychological Consortium - DBT Consultation Team. DBT Bulletin, 5(11), 17–19.

Greville-Harris, M., Hempel, R., Karl, A., Dieppe, P., & Lynch, T. R. (2016). The power of invalidating communication: Receiving invalidating feedback predicts threat-related emotional, physiological, and social responses. *Journal of Social and Clinical Psychology, 35*(6), 471–493.

Grove, J., & Crowell, S. E. (2018). A developmental biosocial model of borderline personality disorder. In J. J. Gross (Ed.), *Handbook of emotion regulation* (2nd ed., pp. 465–480). Guilford Press.

Guarda, A. S., Hanson, A., Mehler, P., & Westmoreland, P. (2022). Terminal anorexia nervosa is a dangerous term: It cannot, and should not, be defined. *Journal of Eating Disorders, 10*(1), 79.

Hall, K. D., Astrachan-Fletcher, E., & Simic, M. (2022). *The radically open DBT workbook for eating disorders: From overcontrol and loneliness to recovery and connection*. New Harbinger.

Hambleton, A., Pepin, G., Le, A., Maloney, D., Aouad, P., Touyz, S., & Maguire, S. (2022). Psychiatric and medical comorbidities of eating disorders: Findings from a rapid review of the literature. *Journal of Eating Disorders, 10*(1), 132.

Harned, M. S. (2022). *Treating trauma in dialectical behavior therapy: The DBT prolonged exposure protocol (DBT PE)*. Guilford Press.

Harrison, A., O'Brien, N., Lopez, C., & Treasure, J. (2010). Sensitivity to reward and punishment in eating disorders. *Psychiatry Research, 177*(1–2), 1–11.

Harrison, A., Sullivan, S., Tchanturia, K., & Treasure, J. (2010). Emotional functioning in eating disorders: Attentional bias, emotion recognition and emotion regulation. *Psychological Medicine, 40*(11), 1887–1897.

Heard, H. L., & Swales, M. A. (2015). *Changing behavior in DBT: Problem solving in action*. Guilford Press.

Hempel, R., Vanderbleek, E., & Lynch, T. R. (2018). Radically open dialectical behavior therapy: Targeting emotional loneliness in anorexia nervosa. *Behaviour Research and Therapy, 110,* 30–37.

Herpertz-Dahlmann, B. (2021). Intensive treatments in adolescent anorexia nervosa. *Nutrients, 13*(4), 1265.

Hewitt, P. L., Flett, G. L., & Ediger, E. (1995). Perfectionism traits and perfectionistic self-presentation in eating disorder attitudes, characteristics, and symptoms. *International Journal of Eating Disorders, 18*(4), 317–326.

Huryk, K. M., Drury, C. R., & Loeb, K. L. (2021). Diseases of affluence? A systematic review of the literature on socioeconomic diversity in eating disorders. *Eating Behaviors, 43,* 101548.

Ingrosso, G., Nisticò, V., Lombardi, F., Chiudinelli, E., Bianchini, G., Faggioli, R., et al. (2024). Autistic traits, sensory sensitivity and eating disturbances in a sample of young adults referring to a generalized mental health clinic. *Eating and Weight Disorders—Studies on Anorexia, Bulimia and Obesity, 29(*1), 10.

Isaksson, M., Ghaderi, A., Wolf-Arehult, M., Öster, C., & Ramklint, M. (2021). Sharing and connecting with others - patient experiences of radically open dialectical behavior therapy for anorexia nervosa and overcontrol: A qualitative study. *Journal of Eating Disorders, 9*(1), 29.

Johns, G., Taylor, B., John, A., & Tan, J. (2019). Current eating disorder healthcare services: The perspectives and experiences of individuals with eating disorders, their families and health professionals: Systematic review and thematic synthesis. *BJPsych Open, 5*(4), e59.

Joiner, T. E., Jr, Brown, J. S., & Wingate, L. R. (2005). The psychology and neurobiology of suicidal behavior. *Annual Review of Psychology, 56,* 287–314.

Kazdin, A. E., Fitzsimmons-Craft, E. E., & Wilfley, D. E. (2017). Addressing critical gaps in the treatment of eating disorders. *International Journal of Eating Disorders, 50*(3), 170–189.

Kliem, S., Kröger, C., & Kosfelder, J. (2010). Dialectical behavior therapy for borderline personality disorder: A meta-analysis using mixed-effects modeling. *Journal of Consulting and Clinical Psychology, 78*(6), 936–951.

Koerner, K. (2011). *Doing dialectical behavior therapy: A practical guide.* Guilford Press.

Kramer, A. M., Smith, J. L., & Johnson, R. D. (2024). Reducing anti-fat bias toward the self and others: A randomized controlled trial. *Journal of Eating Disorders, 12,* Article 46.

Kröger, C., Schweiger, U., Sipos, V., Kliem, S., Arnold, R., Schunert, T., & Reinecker, H. (2010). Dialectical behaviour therapy and an added cognitive behavioural treatment module for eating disorders in women with borderline personality disorder and anorexia nervosa or bulimia nervosa who failed to respond to previous treatments. An open trial with a 15-month follow-up. *Journal of Behavior Therapy and Experimental Psychiatry, 41*(4), 381–388.

Lawrence, B. J., Kerr, D., Pollard, C. M., Theophilus, M., Alexander, E., Haywood, D., & O'Connor, M. (2021). Weight bias among health care professionals: A systematic review and meta-analysis. *Obesity, 29(*11), 1802–1812.

Liakopoulou, E., Vassalou, G., Tzavara, C., & Gonidakis, F. (2023). A 12-month study of dialectical behavioral therapy for borderline patients suffering from eating disorders. *Eating and Weight Disorders, 28*(1), 81.

Limbrunner, H. M., Ben-Porath, D. D., & Wisniewski, L. (2011). DBT telephone skills coaching with eating disordered clients: Who calls, for what reasons, and for how long? *Cognitive and Behavioral Practice, 18*(2), 186–195.

Linardon, J., Wade, T. D., de la Piedad Garcia, X., & Brennan, L. (2017). The efficacy of cognitive-behavioral therapy for eating disorders: A systematic review and meta-analysis. *Journal of Consulting and Clinical Psychology, 85*(11), 1080–1094.

Linehan, M. M. (1993). *Cognitive-behavioral treatment of borderline personality disorder.* Guilford Press.

Linehan, M. M. (1997). Validation and psychotherapy. In A. C. Bohart & L. S. Greenberg (Eds.), *Empathy reconsidered: New directions in psychotherapy* (pp. 353–392). American Psychological Association.

Linehan, M. M. (2025a). *DBT skills training manual* (rev. ed.). Guilford Press.

Linehan, M. M. (2025b). *DBT skills training handouts and worksheets* (rev. ed.). Guilford Press..

Little, J. N., & Codd, R. T., 3rd (2020). Radically Open Dialectical Behavior Therapy (RO DBT) in the treatment of perfectionism: A case study. *Journal of Clinical Psychology, 76*(11), 2097–2108.

Lock, J., & Le Grange, D. (2013). *Treatment manual for anorexia nervosa: A family-based approach* (2nd ed.). Guilford Press.

Lock, J., Le Grange, D., Agras, W. S., Moye, A., Bryson, S. W., & Jo, B. (2010). Randomized clinical trial comparing family-based treatment with adolescent-focused individual therapy for adolescents with anorexia nervosa. *Archives of General Psychiatry, 67*(10), 1025–1032.

Lubieniecki, G., Fernando, A. N., Randhawa, A., Cowlishaw, S., & Sharpe, G. (2024). Perceived clinician stigma and its impact on eating disorder treatment experiences: A systematic review of the lived experience literature. *Journal of Eating Disorders, 12*(1), 161.

Lungu, A., & Linehan, M. M. (2016). Dialectical behavior therapy: A comprehensive multi- and transdiagnostic intervention. In C. M. Nezu & A. M. Nezu (Eds.), *The Oxford handbook of cognitive and behavioral therapies* (pp. 200–214). Oxford University Press.

Lynch, T. R., Gray, K. L., Hempel, R. J., Titley, M., Chen, E. Y., & O'Mahen, H. A. (2013). Radically open-dialectical behavior therapy for adult anorexia nervosa: Feasibility and outcomes from an inpatient program. *BMC Psychiatry, 13*, 293.

Madden, S., Miskovic-Wheatley, J., Wallis, A., Kohn, M., Hay, P., & Touyz, S. (2015). Early weight gain in family-based treatment predicts greater weight gain and remission at the end of treatment and remission at 12-month follow-up in adolescent anorexia nervosa. *International Journal of Eating Disorders, 48*(7), 919–922.

Marek, R. J., Ben-Porath, D. D., Federici, A., Wisniewski, L., & Warren, M. (2013). Targeting premeal anxiety in eating disordered clients and normal controls: A preliminary investigation into the use of mindful eating vs. distraction during food exposure. *International Journal of Eating Disorders, 46*, 582–585.

Marino, J., Hardin, R., Gasbarro, A., Dansereau, V. A., & Fischer, S. (2020). Outpatient treatment for adults with complex eating disorders and co-morbid conditions: A decision making model and case example. *Eating Disorders, 28*(2), 171–183.

Martinelli, M. K., Schreyer, C. C., Vanzhula, I. A., & Guarda, A. S. (2024). Impulsivity and reward and punishment sensitivity among patients admitted to a specialized inpatient eating disorder treatment program. *Frontiers in Psychiatry, 15,* 1325252.

Masson, P. C., von Ranson, K. M., Wallace, L. M., & Safer, D. L. (2013). A randomized wait-list controlled pilot study of dialectical behaviour therapy guided self-help for binge eating disorder. *Behaviour Research and Therapy, 51*(11), 723–728.

Mastria, G., Mancini, V., Viganò, A., & Di Piero, V. (2016). Alice in Wonderland syndrome: A clinical and pathophysiological review. *BioMed Research International, 2016,* 8243145.

Mastria, G., Mancini, V., Di Cesare, M., Puma, M., Alessiani, M., Petolicchio, B., et al. (2021). Prevalence and characteristics of Alice in Wonderland syndrome in adult migraineurs: Perspectives from a tertiary referral headache unit. *Cephalalgia, 41*(5), 515–524.

McColl, C., Hindle, S., & Donkin, L. (2024). *"I mean, it kind of saved my life, to be honest": A qualitative study of participants' views of dialectical behaviour therapy for Multiproblematic Eating Disorders Group Programme.* Research Square.

Meyer-Lindenberg, A., Buckholtz, J. W., Kolachana, B., Hariri, A. R., Pezawas, L., Blasi, G., et al. (2006). Neural mechanisms of genetic risk for impulsivity and violence in humans. *Proceedings of the National Academy of Sciences, 103*(16), 6269–6274.

Mitchison, D., & Hay, P. J. (2014). The epidemiology of eating disorders: Genetic, environmental, and societal factors. *Clinical Epidemiology, 6*, 89–97.

Murphy, R., Straebler, S., Cooper, Z., & Fairburn, C. G. (2010). Cognitive behavioral therapy for eating disorders. *Psychiatric Clinics of North America, 33*(3), 611–627.

Navarro-Haro, M.V., Botella, C., Guillen, V. et al. Dialectical Behavior Therapy in the Treatment of Borderline Personality Disorder and Eating Disorders Comorbidity: A Pilot Study in a Naturalistic Setting. Cogn Ther Res 42, 636–649 (2018).

Navarro-Haro, M. V., Modrego-Alarcón, M., Hoffman, H. G., López-Montoyo, A., Navarro-Gil, M., Montero-Marin, J., et al. (2019). Evaluation of a mindfulness-based intervention with and without virtual reality dialectical behavior therapy® mindfulness skills training for the treatment of generalized anxiety disorder in primary care: A pilot study. *Frontiers in Psychology, 10,* 55.

Niedtfeld, I., & Bohus, M. (2018). Understanding the bio in the biosocial theory of BPD: Recent developments and implications for treatment. In M. A. Swales (Ed.), *The Oxford handbook of dialectical behaviour therapy* (pp. 23–46). Oxford University Press.

Nowakowski, M. E., McFarlane, T., & Cassin, S. (2013). Alexithymia and eating disorders: A critical review of the literature. *Journal of Eating Disorders, 1*(1), 21.

Nunn, K., Frampton, I., Gordon, I., & Lask, B. (2008). The fault is not in her parents but in her insula—A neurobiological hypothesis of anorexia nervosa. *European Eating Disorders Review, 16*(5), 355–360.

Ochsner, K. N., & Gross, J. J. (2014). The neural bases of emotion and emotion regulation: A valuation perspective. In J. J. Gross (Ed.), *Handbook of emotion regulation* (2nd ed., pp. 23–42). Guilford Press.

Oliverio, S., Steiger, H., St-Hilaire, A., Paquin-Hodge, C., Leloup, A. G., Israel, M., & Thaler, L. (2022). Barriers and facilitators to providing autonomy supportive counselling to individuals seeking treatment for an eating disorder. *Eating and Weight Disorders: EWD, 27*(7), 2919–2929.

Palmer, R. L., Birchall, H., Damani, S., Gatward, N., McGrain, L., & Parker, L. (2003). A dialectical behavior therapy program for people with an eating disorder and borderline personality disorder: Description and outcome. *International Journal of Eating Disorders, 33*(3), 281–286.

Pennell, A., Webb, C., Agar, P., Federici, A., & Couturier, J. (2019). Implementation of dialectical behavior therapy in a day hospital setting for adolescents with eating disorders. *Journal of the Canadian Academy of Child & Adolescent Psychiatry, 28*(1), 21.

Pitron, V., Alsmith, A., & de Vignemont, F. (2018). How do the body schema and the body image interact? *Consciousness and Cognition, 65,* 352–358.

Rahmani, M., Omidi, A., Asemi, Z., & Akbari, H. (2018). The effect of dialectical behaviour therapy on binge eating, difficulties in emotion regulation and BMI in overweight patients with binge-eating disorder: A randomized controlled trial. *Mental Health and Prevention, 9,* 13–18.

Ralph, A. F., Brennan, L., Byrne, S., Caldwell, B., Farmer, J., Hart, L. M., et al. (2022). Management of eating disorders for people with higher weight: Clinical practice guideline. *Journal of Eating Disorders, 10*(1), 121.

Rathus, J. H., & Miller, A. L. (2000). DBT for adolescents: Dialectical dilemmas and secondary treatment targets. *Cognitive and Behavioral Practice,* 7(4), 425–434.

Reay, M., Holliday, J., Stewart, J., & Adams, J. (2022). Creating a care pathway for patients with longstanding, complex eating disorders. *Journal of Eating Disorders, 10*(1), 128.

Rizvi, S. L. (2019). *Chain analysis in dialectical behavior therapy.* Guilford Press.

Rossier, V., Bolognini, M., Plancherel, B., & Halfon, O. (2000). Sensation seeking: A personality trait characteristic of adolescent girls and young women with eating disorders? *European Eating Disorder Review, 8*(3), 245–252.

Safer, D. L., Adler, S., & Masson, P. C. (2018). *The DBT solution for emotional eating: A proven program to break the cycle of bingeing and out-of-control eating*. Guilford Press.

Safer, D. L., Telch, C. F., & Chen, E. Y. (2017). *Dialectical behavior therapy for binge eating and bulimia*. Guilford Press.

Safer, D. L., Telch, C. F., & Agras, W. S. (2001a). Dialectical behavior therapy adapted for bulimia: A case report. *International Journal of Eating Disorders, 30*(1), 101–106.

Safer, D. L., Telch, C. F., & Chen, E. Y. (2009). *Dialectical behavior therapy for binge eating and bulimia*. Guilford Press.

Salbach-Andrae, H., Bohnekamp, I., Pfeiffer, E., Lehmkuhl, U., & Miller, A. L. (2008). Dialectical behavior therapy of anorexia and bulimia nervosa among adolescents: A case series. *Cognitive and Behavioral Practice, 15*(4), 415–425.

Sayrs, J. H. R., & Linehan, M. M. (2019). *DBT teams: Development and practice*. Guilford Press.

Seah, X. Y., Tham, X. C., Kamaruzaman, N. R., & Yobas, P. (2017). Knowledge, attitudes and challenges of healthcare professionals managing people with eating disorders: A literature review. *Archives of Psychiatric Nursing, 31*(1), 125–136.

Sharpe S. L. (2024). A living experience proposal for the co-occurring diagnosis of avoidant/restrictive food intake disorder and other eating disorders. *Journal of Eating Disorders, 12*(1), 110.

Shenk, C. E., & Fruzzetti, A. E. (2011). The impact of validating and invalidating responses on emotional reactivity. *Journal of Social and Clinical Psychology, 30*(2), 163–185.

Sonneville, K. R., & Lipson, S. K. (2018). Disparities in eating disorder diagnosis and treatment according to weight status, race/ethnicity, socioeconomic background, and sex among college students. *International Journal of Eating Disorders, 51*(6), 518–526.

Stice, E., Marti, C. N., Spoor, S., Presnell, K., & Shaw, H. (2008). Dissonance and healthy weight eating disorder prevention programs: Long-term effects from a randomized efficacy trial. *Journal of Consulting and Clinical Psychology, 76*(2), 329–340.

Strings, S. (2019). *Fearing the black body: The racial origins of fat phobia*. New York University Press.

Swenson, C. R. (2016). *DBT principles in action: Acceptance, change, and dialectics*. Guilford Press.

Tchanturia, K., Davies, H., & Campbell, I. C. (2007). Cognitive remediation therapy for patients with anorexia nervosa: Preliminary findings. *Annals of General Psychiatry, 6*(1), Article 14.

Tchanturia, K., Davies, H., Roberts, M., Harrison, A., Nakazato, M., Schmidt, U., & Treasure, J. (2012). Poor cognitive flexibility in eating disorders: Examining the evidence using the Wisconsin Card Sorting Task. *PLoS ONE, 7*(1), e28331.

Tchanturia, K., Larsson, E., & Adamson, J. (2016). Brief group intervention targeting cognitive and emotional functioning in eating disorders: A pilot study. *Eating and Weight Disorders—Studies on Anorexia, Bulimia and Obesity, 21*(1), 107–113.

Termorshuizen, J. D., Davies, H. L., Lee, S. H., Huckins, L. M., Bulik, C. M., Breen, G., et al. (2025). Genome-wide association studies of binge-eating behaviour and anorexia nervosa yield insights into the unique and shared biology of eating disorder phenotypes. *medRxiv,* 2025.01.31.25321397.

Thomas, C., Claudat, K.., Hindle, S., & Federici, A. (2024, July). What happens next? The principles and practicalities of treating stage II clients with multi-problem eating disorders. *DBT Bulletin, 8*(1), 37–41.

Thomas, E., Russell, J., & Touyz, S. (2024). Neurodivergence, intersectionality, and eating disorders: A lived experience-led narrative review. *Journal of Eating Disorders, 12*(1), 74.

Thomas, J. J., & Gydus, J. E. (2023). A proposed trumping scheme for other specified feeding or eating disorder: Comment on Walsh et al., 2023. *The International Journal of Eating Disorders, 56*(4), 835–837.

Thompson-Brenner, H., Satir, D. A., Franko, D. L., & Herzog, D. B. (2012). Clinicians reactions to patients with eating disorders: A review of the literature. *Psychiatric Services, 63*(1), 73–78.

Touyz, S., Bryant, E., Dann, K. M., Polivy, J., Le Grange, D., Hay, P., et al. (2023). What kind of illness is anorexia nervosa? Revisited: Some preliminary thoughts to finding a cure. *Journal of Eating Disorders, 11,* 221.

Treasure, J., & Schmidt, U. (2013). The cognitive-interpersonal maintenance model of anorexia nervosa revisited: A summary of the evidence for cognitive, socio-emotional, and interpersonal predisposing and perpetuating factors. *Journal of Eating Disorders, 1*(1), 13.

Treasure, J., Willmott, D., Ambwani, S., Cardi, V., Clark Bryan, D., Rowlands, K., & Schmidt, U. (2020). Cognitive interpersonal model for Anorexia Nervosa revisited: The Perpetuating factors that contribute to the development of the severe and enduring illness. *Journal of Clinical Medicine, 9*(3), 630.

Tse, A., Xavier, S., Trollope-Kumar, K., Agarwal, G., & Lokker, C. (2022). Challenges in eating disorder diagnosis and management among family physicians and trainees: A qualitative study. *Journal of Eating Disorders, 10,* 45.

Uher, R., Murphy, T., Friederich, H.-C., Dalgleish, T., Brammer, M. J., Giampietro, V., et al. (2005). Functional neuroanatomy of body shape perception in healthy and eating-disordered women. *Biological Psychiatry, 58*(12), 990–997.

Vinchenzo, C., Lawrence, V., & McCombie, C. (2022). Patient perspectives on premature termination of eating disorder treatment: A systematic review and qualitative synthesis. *Journal of Eating Disorders, 10*(1), Article 39.

Waller, G., Cordery, H., Corstorphine, E., Hinrichsen, H., Lawson, R., Mountford, V., & Russell, K. (2007). *Cognitive behavioral therapy for eating disorders: A comprehensive treatment guide.* Cambridge University Press.

Watson, H. J., Yilmaz, Z., Thornton, L. M., Hübel, C., Coleman, J. R. I., Gaspar, H. A., et al. (2019). Genome-wide association study identifies eight risk loci and implicates metabo-psychiatric origins for anorexia nervosa. *Nature Genetics, 51*(8), 1207–1214.

Westwood, H., Mandy, W., Simic, M., & Tchanturia, K. (2017). The association between symptoms of autism and neuropsychological performance in females with anorexia nervosa. *European Eating Disorders Review, 25*(2), 123–130.

Wilson, G. T., Grilo, C. M., & Vitousek, K. M. (2007). Psychological treatment of eating disorders. *American Psychologist, 62*(3), 199–216.

Wisniewski, L., & Ben-Porath, D. D. (2005). Telephone skill-coaching with eating-disordered clients: Clinical guidelines using a DBT framework. *European Eating Disorders Review, 13*(5), 344–350.

Wisniewski, L., & Ben-Porath, D. D. (2015). Dialectical behavior therapy and eating disorders: The use of contingency management procedures to manage dialectical dilemmas. *American Journal of Psychotherapy, 69*(2), 129–140.

Wisniewski, L., & Kelly, E. (2003). The application of dialectical behavior therapy to the treatment of eating disorders. *Cognitive and Behavioral Practice, 10*(2), 131–138.

Wisniewski, L., Safer, D. L., & Chen, E. Y. (2007). Dialectical behavior therapy and eating disorders. In L. Dimeff & K. Koerner (Eds.), *Dialectical behavior therapy in clinical practice: Applications across disorders and settings* (pp. 174–221). Guilford Press.

Zhao, J., Zhang, R., & Feng, T. (2024). Relationship between punishment sensitivity and risk-taking propensity. *Brain and Cognition, 181*, 106222.

Zucker, N., Le Grange, D., & Muench, F. (2007). Anorexia nervosa and autism spectrum disorders: Guided investigation of social cognitive endophenotypes. *Psychological Bulletin, 133*(6), 1018–1034.

# Index